AUTOIMMUNE PROTOCOL JUICING COOKBOOK FOR SENIORS

(AIP)

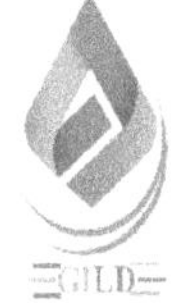

AUTOIMMUNE PROTOCOL JUICING COOKBOOK FOR SENIORS

Natural Recipes for Body Nourishment, Anti-Aging, Chronic Disease Prevention, Inflammation Reduction, Weight Loss, Energy Boost, Detoxification, Enhanced Immune System, and Improved Gut Health

Lilian Daniel

Copyright

Disclaimer

This publication is designed to provide competent and reliable information regarding the subject matter covered. However, it is sold with the understanding that the author is not engaged in rendering professional or nutritional advice. Laws and practices often vary from state to state and country to country and if medical or other expert assistance is required, the service of a professional should be sought.

Table of Contents

Introduction

I'm thrilled and delighted that you're here. If you're reading this, you're likely on a journey to free your body and mind from the grip of an autoimmune illness. I know firsthand how daunting and isolating this can feel. But I want you to know that you're not alone, and there is hope for a vibrant healthy life, free from the constraints of chronic illness.

I still remember 27 years ago, the gentle sway of the boat on the tranquil waters of river Guadalupe in Texas, surrounded by the quiet countryside. I was sitting side by side with a Friend's dad in a sturdy fishing boat, the early morning sunlight casting a golden glow on the rippling surface of the water.

we both cast our lines into the river, the anticipation of a bite hangs in the air. Suddenly, Dr Charles, my friend's dad felts a tug on his line. With a grin of excitement, he starts reeling in the catch. As he leans back slightly to gain leverage, he lets out a small sigh, acknowledging the familiar ache in his back.

"Ah, my back's acting up a bit," he admits with a chuckle, turning to me. "Could you lend me a hand with this?"

I reached over to support him, sharing in the effort of pulling the fish closer to the boat. With a triumphant grin, he finally lands the fish onto the deck.

"Sir, you're not as young as you used to be," I teased gently, handing him the rod.

He laughs good-naturedly, nodding in agreement. "You got me there, kiddo. But hey, age doesn't stop me from enjoying moments like this with you."

As seniors age will never stop you from being young, aging is a natural process, but it doesn't define one's capacity for joy or adventure. Reflecting on this, you might draw a parallel to the principles of maintaining vitality and wellness, such as those, that are outlined in this book. Following a protocol that supports well-being, whether through nutrition, exercise, or mindset, can empower you to embrace each day with energy and optimism.

This book is important and beneficial to you, if you are seeking to take a proactive approach to managing your health, particularly if you have autoimmune issues or want to optimize your immune system. It offers a roadmap for incorporating nutrient-dense, healing foods into your diet through delicious and easy-to-prepare juice recipes.

Understanding The Root-Cause

As we age, the immune system undergoes various changes that contributes to an increased risk of autoimmune problems. To understand why we are more susceptible to autoimmune disorders, it's important to understand the complex interplay of immunological alterations and other factors associated with aging.

Don't be surprise when you can't do the simple daily things, you find so easily to do. Our body system response in various ways as we age. Autoimmune disorders occur when the immune system, which normally protects the body from harmful substances like bacteria and viruses, mistakenly attacks healthy cells and tissues.

This led to a wide range of conditions such as rheumatoid arthritis, lupus, type 1 diabetes, and multiple sclerosis, among other. One of the key reasons seniors are more prone to autoimmune disorders is a phenomenon called immunosenescence, which refers to the gradual decline in immune function that comes with aging.

As we age, our immune system becomes less efficient and less capable of distinguishing between self and non-self-antigens. Which in most cases increases the likelihood of autoimmunity.

Factors and Reasons why Seniors Are Prone to Autoimmune Problems.

1. **Changes in T Cells**

- T cells (are a specific kind of white blood cell known as lymphocytes. They play a crucial role in helping the immune system combat germs and diseases). With age, the diversity of T cells decreases, and their ability to respond to new pathogens diminishes. Moreover, there is a shift towards more memory T cells, which could contribute to the development of autoimmune diseases as these cells may become activated inappropriately against self-antigens.

2. **Decreased B Cell Regulation**

- B cells are also a type of white blood cell, specifically lymphocytes, their role is critical in the immune system's defense against infections. These cells are responsible for producing antibodies, which are proteins that can recognize and neutralize specific invaders like bacteria, viruses, and other harmful substances. As we age, the regulatory mechanisms that control B cell activity can become impaired. This loss of control result in the production of excessive or inappropriate antibodies. Which may/may not contribute to the development or exacerbation of autoimmune conditions commonly seen in seniors. B cells interact closely with T cells in orchestrating immune responses.

3. **Chronic Inflammation**

   As we age, our bodies may experience inflammation, which is a normal response to injury or infection. This process helps us heal and stay healthy by sending special chemicals and white blood cells to the affected area is called acute inflammation and can usually last a few hours to a few days.

   However, sometimes this inflammation doesn't go away easily and may become chronic. Chronic inflammation can be harmful, causing pain, discomfort, and limiting our mobility. It can affect different parts of our body and may lead to other health issues.

Chronic inflammation in seniors is a long-term, low-grade immune system response that persists even when there is no apparent threat or infection. It's like the body's alarm system being stuck in the "on" position.

While inflammation is a normal and necessary process for fighting off infections and promoting healing, chronic inflammation is different because it lingers for extended periods, potentially causing harm to tissues and organs.

As we get older (Seniors), we often have chronic medical conditions such as cardiovascular disease, diabetes, arthritis, and autoimmune disorders, which can sustain inflammation. Inflammation is both a cause and consequence of these conditions, creating a vicious cycle.

Causes of Chronic Inflammation in Seniors

Accumulated Wear and Tear: Over time, our body undergoes natural wear and tear, leading to cellular damage and the release of inflammatory molecules. The wear-and-tear theory of aging suggests that as we age, our bodies experience gradual damage to cells and systems from years of use.

This theory proposes that our bodies "wear out" over time, much like a machine that becomes less effective with frequent use.

Eventually, this accumulated wear and tear can lead to a decline in the body's ability to function properly.

Causes of Wear-and-Tear Damage: Various factors, both internal and external, can harm our body systems. Exposure to radiation, toxins, and ultraviolet light can damage our genes. Also, the body's own processes, such as oxygen metabolism, produce free radicals that can cause damage to our cells and tissues.

Certain cellular systems in our bodies, like the nerve cells in the brain, do not replace themselves over our lifetime. When these cells are lost, it can lead to a decline in their function over time.

In cells, that keep dividing DNA can suffer damage and accumulate errors over time. The repetitive division process gradually shortens the telomeres at the ends of chromosomes, eventually leading to cells that can no longer divide (senescent cells). Additionally, oxidative damage within cells causes proteins to cross-link, hindering their proper function. Free radicals generated inside mitochondria, which are the energy producers of cells, can also damage their membranes, impairing their efficiency.

Poor Diet: Diets high in processed foods, sugars, and unhealthy fats can contribute to inflammation. While a poor diet may not directly cause autoimmune diseases, it can influence the severity and timing of symptoms. Malnutrition or a diet lacking essential nutrients can impair the production and function of immune cells and antibodies. Also, poor digestion can contribute to the formation of antigens that trigger autoimmune reactions. For instance, in celiac disease, gluten intolerance prompts an immune response against the lining of the small intestine.

Smoking: Tobacco smoke contains toxins that trigger inflammation in the body. In addition to its well-known associations with cancer, lung diseases, and cardiovascular diseases, smoking profoundly affects the immune system. It elevates inflammation levels, heightens the likelihood of allergic conditions, raises the occurrence of autoimmune diseases, diminishes immune responses to infectious diseases, and boosts infection rates.

Cigarette smoke initiates inflammation by stimulating an inflammatory response, affecting both the lungs and the entire body. The chemicals in cigarette smoke interact with different types of immune cells, causing an increase in the number of cells gathering at the site of inflammation. This interaction also alters the levels of cytokines (signaling molecules released by immune cells) and other biological substances that control inflammation.

Impact of Chronic Inflammation in Seniors

Increased Risk of Chronic Diseases: Chronic inflammation is associated with various age-related diseases, including heart disease, diabetes, arthritis, and neurodegenerative disorders like Alzheimer's disease.

Weakened Immune Function: Prolonged inflammation can impair the immune system's ability to function properly, making seniors more susceptible to infections.

Joint and Muscle Pain: Inflammation in the joints (arthritis) and muscles can cause pain and stiffness, reducing mobility and quality of life. Rheumatoid arthritis is an autoimmune disease that causes inflammation, pain, swelling, stiffness, and loss of function in the joints. It typically affects synovial joints in the hands, arms, knees, and feet. Many us with rheumatoid arthritis experience significant fatigue, which can make it challenging to participate fully in daily activities.

Cognitive Decline: Chronic inflammation is implicated in cognitive decline and may contribute to the development of dementia.

Accelerated Aging: Persistent inflammation is thought to accelerate the aging process at the cellular level, contributing to age-related degeneration.

Managing Chronic Inflammation in Seniors

Healthy Diet: Emphasize a balanced diet rich in fruits, vegetables, whole grains, and healthy fats (e.g., omega-3 fatty acids)

Regular Exercise: Engage in regular physical activity to reduce inflammation and improve overall health.

Weight Management: Maintain a healthy weight to reduce inflammation associated with obesity.

Smoking Cessation: Quit smoking to decrease inflammation and improve overall health.

Stress Management: Practice stress-reducing techniques such as meditation, yoga, or deep breathing exercises.

Medication: In some cases, medication may be prescribed to control inflammation and manage symptoms of inflammatory conditions.

4. Environmental Exposures

- Exposure to environmental dust has been linked to the advancement of autoimmune diseases. This connection involves several mechanisms, such as systemic inflammation, increased oxidative stress, changes in gene regulation (epigenetic alterations), and immune responses triggered by damage to the airways. Prolonged exposure to air pollution is associated with an increased likelihood of autoimmune diseases, particularly rheumatoid arthritis, connective tissue disorders, and inflammatory bowel diseases.
  Several environmental factors that might aid these autoimmune diseases (Ads) include:

Air Pollution: Long-term exposure to air pollution from vehicle exhaust and industrial emissions can activate the body's adaptive immune response, potentially leading to tissue damage and inflammation. Particulate matter in air pollution can also induce oxidative stress and cell death, exacerbating chronic inflammation.

External factors: such as drugs, chemicals, microbes, and other environmental elements can trigger autoimmunity, particularly systemic autoimmune diseases. To elaborate, certain drugs or chemicals prompts an immune response that mistakenly targets the body's own tissues.

For example, certain medications can cause drug-induced lupus, where the immune system attacks healthy cells in a similar manner to systemic lupus erythematosus (SLE) but usually resolves once the medication is stopped. Microbes like bacteria or viruses can also stimulate immune responses that cross-react with self-antigens, leading to autoimmune reactions.

5. **Genetic Predisposition**

As we get older each day, certain diseases develop due to genetic traits that were once beneficial during youth but become less helpful with age. Longevity is linked to having a robust natural immune system. The aging of the immune system, known as immunosenescence, is affected by ongoing exposure to chronic antigens like infections.

This is why living longer is more likely in environments with fewer pathogens. Lower pathogen exposure helps maintain a balanced immune response and reduces the risk of developing severe inflammatory reactions.

Autoimmune diseases often cluster within families, a phenomenon known as "familial aggregation." The likelihood of a specific autoimmune disease occurring in identical twins (with a concordance rate typically ranging from 25% to 50%) is significantly higher compared to fraternal twins (with a concordance rate typically ranging from 2% to 8%). These findings highlight a strong genetic influence on autoimmune diseases.

Inheritance can play a role in autoimmune disorders, but several other factors are also involved. While the exact causes of autoimmune diseases are not fully understood, family history is known to influence susceptibility. DNA testing for autoimmune diseases can provide valuable insights into your genetic risk, although it cannot definitively predict whether you will develop specific diseases. Instead, it can indicate whether you have a higher risk compared to the general population.

In many cases, specific autoimmune diseases are not strongly influenced by heredity. However, there are exceptions where different autoimmune diseases can occur within the same family. For example, one family member might have lupus while another has autoimmune hypothyroidism or rheumatoid arthritis.

While genes are significant contributors to autoimmune diseases (AID), they are just part of the puzzle. A person's genetic predisposition (meaning their genes make them susceptible) combined with specific environmental factors can lead to AID development. Evidence suggests that certain genetic variations, when combined with factors like infections, exposure to toxins, medications, lifestyle choices, diet, and stress, can trigger AID.

There isn't a single gene responsible for autoimmune diseases (AID). Instead, a group of genes known as the major histocompatibility complex (MHC) plays a significant role in many AID. The MHC carries instructions for producing various cells and molecules crucial for the immune system. Specific HLA genes within the MHC are strongly linked to certain autoimmune conditions such as Type 1 diabetes, rheumatoid arthritis (RA), multiple sclerosis (MS), and myasthenia gravis. Besides the MHC, numerous genes scattered throughout our DNA influence immune function. Changes in these genes are observed in various autoimmune disorders and involve processes like T cell and B cell regulation, among others.

6. Hormonal Changes

Changes in hormones can impact the onset and severity of autoimmune diseases among seniors. For instance, the hormonal shifts during menopause can raise the likelihood of autoimmune conditions in women after menopause. Nevertheless, research has indicated that several autoimmune diseases decrease in women during menopause, coinciding with lower estrogen levels.

Hormones play a role in regulating the immune system and can contribute to the development of autoimmune diseases. Estrogens enhance humoral immunity, whereas androgens and progesterone have natural immunosuppressive effects.

In women of reproductive age, higher estrogen levels often result in a more robust immune response. However, during menopause, the rapid decline in ovarian function and estrogen levels is linked to increased levels of pro-inflammatory cytokines.

In men, reduced androgen levels are linked to conditions like lupus erythematosus (SLE), rheumatoid arthritis (RA), and multiple sclerosis (MS). However, the influence of age-related declines in testosterone on the progression of these diseases are not thoroughly explored.

The impact of hormonal changes in seniors on autoimmune diseases is multifaceted. Decreased levels of estrogen and androgens can have diverse effects, sometimes leading to positive outcomes such as reduced inflammation, while in other cases, they may contribute to negative effects like increased disease activity. The specific impact depends on the type of autoimmune condition.

7. **Cumulative Damage and Stress**

Stressful situations can weaken our body's natural defense system, making us more vulnerable to autoimmune diseases. When we experience ongoing stress, it leads to gut problems like inflammation and leaky gut, which are often linked to autoimmune issues. Long-term stress can mess with our immune system by:

- *Throwing off the balance of different types of immune messengers.*

- *Keeping inflammation going for longer periods.*

- *Weakening the number, movement, and effectiveness of our protective immune cells.*

What is stress?

Stress is commonly understood as any situation that creates tension, whether it's physical, psychological, or emotional. It's the kind of feeling that triggers our body's "fight or flight" response, where the adrenal gland releases adrenaline, causing our heart rate and breathing to speed up, and our blood pressure to rise.

This response is helpful when facing immediate danger, like being chased by a lion. However, ongoing stress, like worrying about finances, health, or relationships, may contribute to chronic conditions such as high blood pressure or autoimmune diseases.

What causes stress varies greatly from person to person. For instance, speaking in public can be a common source of stress. While some of us may find it easy to deliver a speech to a crowd, others may feel intense dread and worry about it for weeks beforehand. There's a significant distinction between general stress and a "stress-related disorder," which refers to a specific condition or disease that develops after a highly stressful event.

A notable example is post-traumatic stress disorder (PTSD), where a severe physical or psychological trauma trigger distressing symptoms like intrusive memories of the event, memory issues, apathy, and irritability.

The Benefits of Natural Juices, Smoothies, and Vegetables Over Medicinal Drugs

It is important to note and acknowledge that natural remedies encompass a wide array of practices and substances derived from plants, herbs, and foods. To be exact, most of the medical drugs are all product of these natural remedies but undergoes a chemical process. Personally, I have six reasons why I choose natural juice to anything out there. Yes! natural juice doesn't always taste sweet and sugary but, the results are always best compared to any drugs.

We are not only going to focus on the recipes alone, but also learning about the health value of these recipes, in my first book: Autoimmune Protocol Juicing Recipes Cookbook (AIP): For Gut Health and Inflammation Relief with Juicing Recipes to Conquer and Combat Autoimmune Challenges and Restore Digestive Wellness, I talked about how eating what you know is freedom and health. So here are my reasons why this book is an exceptional for you.

Targeted Nutrition: Autoimmune protocol (AIP) focuses on specific dietary strategies to help manage autoimmune conditions by reducing inflammation and supporting gut health. this juice book is based on AIP principles and it provides you with recipes and guidance on which ingredients to include (and avoid) to support your body's healing process.

Nutrient Density: Juicing can be an efficient way to consume a concentrated amount of nutrients from fruits, vegetables, and other healing ingredients. This well-designed autoimmune protocol juice book offers recipes that are rich in vitamins, minerals, antioxidants, and phytonutrients, all essential for supporting your immune function and health.

Gut Health Support: The AIP emphasizes foods that promote a healthy gut microbiome, which is crucial for immune regulation and overall wellness. Many autoimmune diseases are linked to gut health, and incorporating gut-healing ingredients into your juices can be beneficial for managing symptoms and improving digestion.

Inflammation Reduction: Chronic inflammation is a common factor in autoimmune conditions. AIP emphasizes anti-inflammatory foods, such as leafy greens, turmeric, ginger, and certain fruits, which can help reduce inflammation and alleviate symptoms associated with autoimmune disorders.

Personalized Approach: this juice book offers a structured approach to discovering which foods work best for your body and which may trigger autoimmune reactions. This personalized approach empowers you to make informed dietary choices that support your unique health needs.

Comprehensive Guidance: Beyond just recipes, we provide educational content on autoimmune diseases, practical tips for implementation, and strategies for lifestyle modifications that complement dietary changes.

This cookbook is Customized for those following the autoimmune protocol, so you can be confident that the recipes are designed to meet your dietary requirements and health goals. Even if you don't have an autoimmune condition, incorporating AIP juicing is a great way to boost your wellness and immune system.

Juicing allows us to consume a larger quantity and variety of fruits and vegetables in an easily digestible form, which ensures we're getting a broad spectrum of nutrients that support optimal health. AIP juicing doesn't have to be bland or boring, so for every recipe, be actively involved.

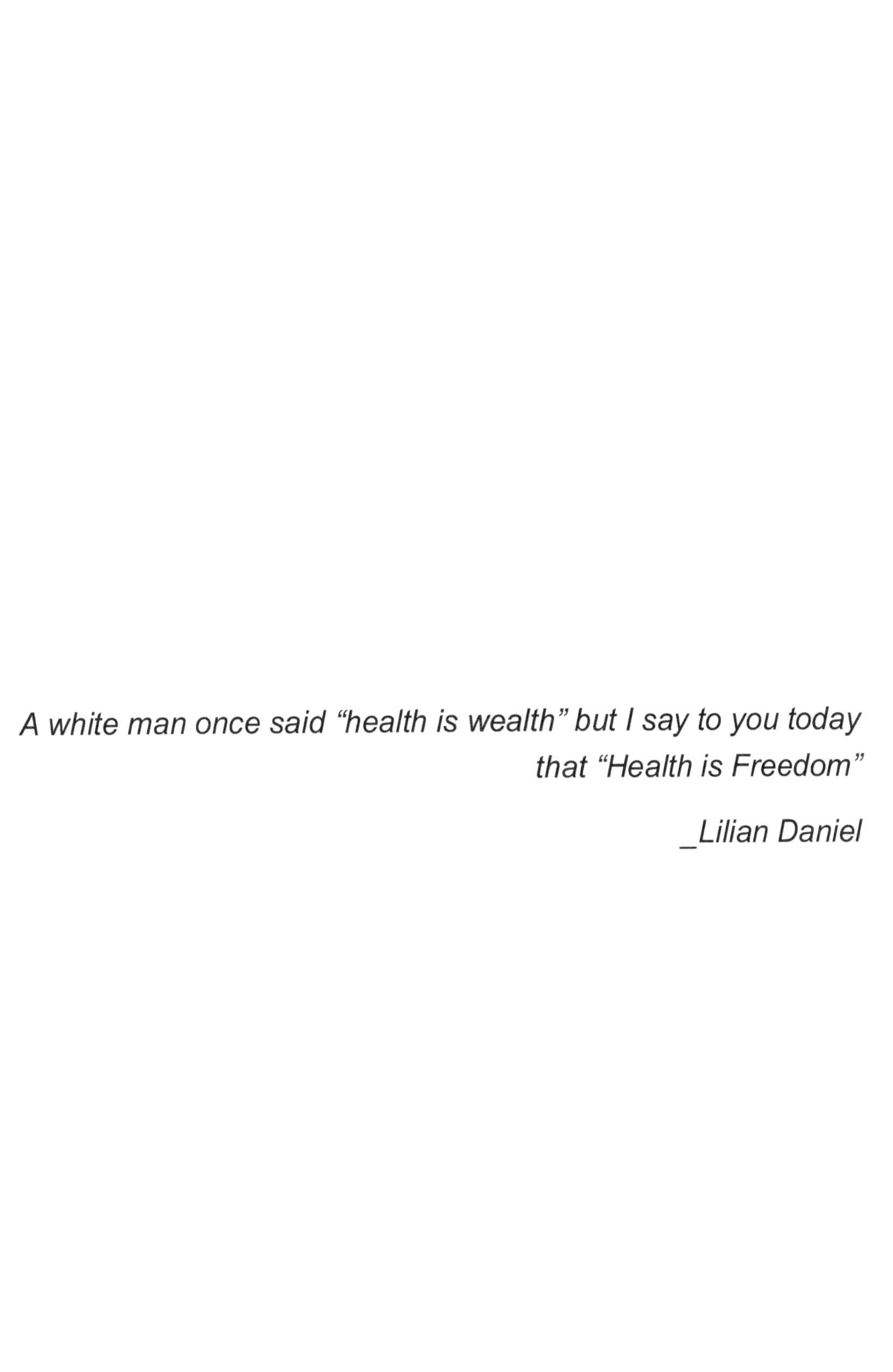

A white man once said "health is wealth" but I say to you today that "Health is Freedom"

_Lilian Daniel

A Better Option Juices or Smoothies

Did you know that the health of your stomach can affect how you feel in general? Experts believe that gut health is connected to many things, like how well you digest food and even how you feel mentally. Eating more fresh fruits and green leafy vegetables can really help our gut health.

Sipping on fruit and vegetable juices is a simple and tasty way to boost your health! It's not only yummy but also offers many benefits, these drinks can make your stomach stronger and help calm inflammation. Juice cleanses, also called juice fasts, mean you only drink freshly squeezed fruit and veggie juices for a set time, usually a few days to a couple of weeks.

Juicing takes out the liquid from fruits and veggies but removes the fiber. Even though fresh juices have lots of vitamins, minerals, and good stuff, they don't have the fiber that's in whole fruits and veggies. Fiber is really important for your digestion and helps keep your blood sugar steady.

On the other hand, smoothies are thick and creamy drinks made by blending different ingredients together in a blender until they're smooth. The best thing about smoothies is that you can put in whatever you like.

Smoothies are different because they keep all the fruit and veggie parts, including the fiber, when they're blended. This fiber makes you feel full, keeps your tummy happy, and helps keep your blood sugar steady. Eating plenty of fiber in your diet can help prevent lots of tummy troubles.

Both fresh juices and smoothies can be good for you, but they affect your health in different ways. Fresh juices have lots of nutrients packed in, but they don't have fiber. Smoothies are a better mix of nutrients and also have fiber. Deciding which one to choose depends on what you want for your health and what you like best.

The most important thing to understand about juice or smoothies is that while in some cases they can help supplement an overall healthy diet, they can't replace eating whole foods.

Natural Juices for Senior Immune Support

EXCLUSIVE ORANGE, CARROT, AND BEET

Juicing is incredibly popular for good reason. When you juice fruits or vegetables, their fibers are removed, leaving behind a concentrated tonic packed with vitamins, minerals, and enzymes that are easily absorbed into our bloodstream. This allows our body to efficiently process the nutrients from fruits and vegetables without putting too much strain on our digestive system.

This Orange, Carrot, and Beet Juice is not only delicious but also visually stunning, thanks to the vibrant beet phytonutrients it contains. With its refreshing and zesty flavors, this juice serves as a delightful pick-me-up.

Freshly squeezed oranges provide a refreshing flavor, complemented by immune-boosting Vitamin A-rich carrots and antioxidant-loaded apples to sweeten the deal. Ginger adds digestive-boosting properties and a spicy kick. The beets shine in this juice, offering detoxifying benefits, iron, Vitamins A, C, & B6, folic acid, and a wealth of other antioxidants.

Beet juice has been demonstrated to lower blood pressure by relaxing and dilating blood vessels in the body. Enjoy this juice with your meal or as a revitalizing afternoon pick-me-up for an energy boost.

RECIPES / INGREDIENTS
2 medium organic beets, scrubbed and roughly chopped
1 bunch of small carrots, chopped (about 6-7 carrots)
1 organic apple, chopped (I used Fuji)
1-inch piece of fresh ginger, peeled
Juice of 6 oranges

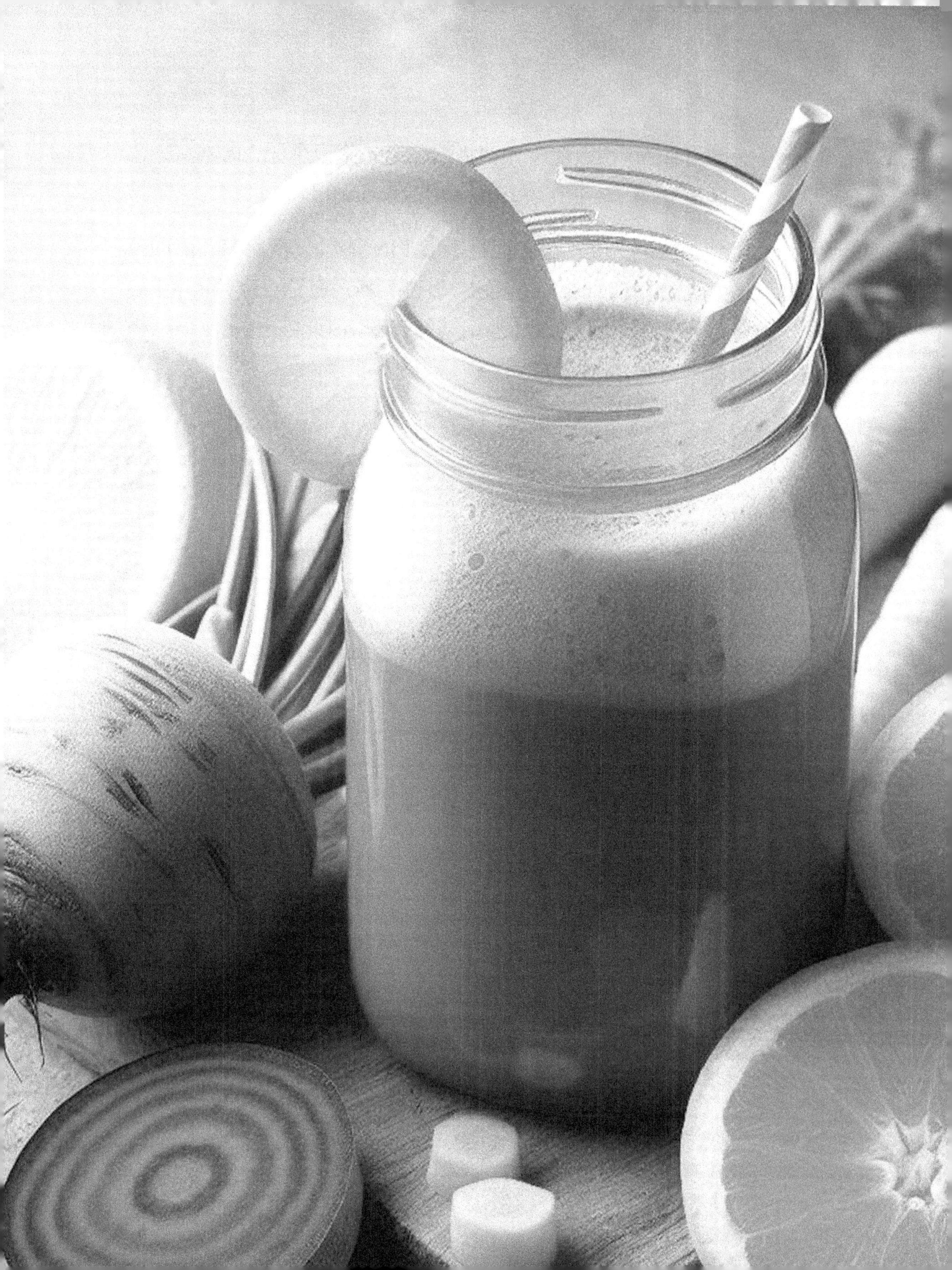

INSTRUCTIONS / DIRECTIONS

In a high-speed blender, combine the juice of 6 oranges with the peeled ginger, chopped apple, carrots, and beets. Blend on high speed for 20-30 seconds until the vegetables and fruits are thoroughly blended and smooth

Strain the blended juice through a nut-milk bag or fine-mesh strainer into a large bowl. Use a rubber spatula or your hands (note: they may be stained temporarily) to press and extract all the juice from the pulp.

Transfer the freshly squeezed juice into a sealed glass container and refrigerate. Enjoy the juice immediately or allow it to chill in the refrigerator. For best quality, consume the juice within 12-24 hours.

If you use your hands to squeeze the pulp and juice through a nut milk bag, your hands will likely become stained red from the beet juice. A thorough scrub with soap and water should remove the stains, but be prepared for temporary discoloration.

Dispose of the pulp by adding it to your compost, or save it for future use in a smoothie. The pulp freezes well and can be a great addition to your next beet-inspired smoothie.

This juice recipe aligns well with the Autoimmune Protocol (AIP) it focuses on nutrient-dense, anti-inflammatory ingredients that support immune health, gut function, and overall wellness. It provides essential vitamins, minerals, antioxidants, and hydration without including common inflammatory triggers, making it a beneficial addition to an AIP-friendly diet.

You can adjust the ingredients according to your taste preferences and dietary needs. If the juice is too thick, add a splash of filtered water to reach your desired consistency and please do not add any sweetener to the juice.

GREEN DETOX

This lively smoothie is a fantastic way to kick off your day. The combination of apple, kiwi, and kale packs a powerful punch of Vitamin C. Each ingredient brings valuable nutrients, and when blended together, they create a dynamo of flavor and health benefits. For the best results, opt for a Granny Smith apple to add a crisp and tangy touch to your smoothie. Enjoy the refreshing taste and nourishing benefits of this vibrant blend.

Some apple varieties are high in sugar and low in antioxidants, but not the Granny Smith. This apple is packed with phytonutrients, most of which are found in the skin. However, since 90% of pesticides are also on the skin, it's important to buy organic and avoid peeling. Kale is another powerhouse, offering impressive levels of Omega-3 fatty acids and Vitamin A. Plus, there's no need to miss milk, as kale provides even more calcium.

Recently, someone asked me, "Aren't you worried about eating goitrogens with autoimmune thyroid disease? My alternative health practitioner told me they could cause a goiter!" Many people are concerned about eating nutritious foods like broccoli, cabbage, sweet potatoes, and strawberries because of this fear.

I'm telling you that eating goitrogens in regular amounts is not harmful if you have autoimmune thyroid disease. In fact, avoiding these foods could deprive you of essential nutrients and do more harm than good. Goitrogens are substances that can interfere with the thyroid's ability to absorb iodine, affecting its function. Besides certain foods, various medications and chemicals also impact this process. Foods known to contain goitrogens include broccoli, Brussels sprouts, cabbage, cauliflower, collard greens, flaxseed, kale, mustard greens, pears, peaches, pine nuts, peanuts, radishes, rutabaga, soy, spinach, strawberries, sweet potatoes, and turnips. While some of these, like flaxseed, pine nuts, peanuts, and soy, are not part of the Autoimmune Protocol (AIP) diet, many others, such as sweet potatoes and cruciferous vegetables, are integral to it.

It's a common myth in the alternative health community that goitrogens cause goiters, which are enlargements of the thyroid gland. However, goiters are not caused by iodine deficiency or eating goitrogens. They are actually caused by inflammation from chronic autoimmune thyroid disease, such as Hashimoto's. To reduce a goiter, you need to address the underlying autoimmune thyroid disease, not eliminate goitrogens from your diet.

Some vegetables classified as goitrogens are also highly nutritious and beneficial to include in our diets. Cruciferous vegetables like broccoli, cabbage, and kale are renowned for their anti-cancer and antioxidant properties. Root vegetables such as sweet potatoes, turnips, and rutabaga are excellent sources of complex carbohydrates, which can be hard to find on a grain-free diet. Cruciferous vegetables, along with sweet potatoes and strawberries, contain carotenoids, which are converted into vitamin A in the body. Many fruits and vegetables on this list are rich in B vitamins, vitamin C, vitamin K, calcium, magnesium, potassium, zinc, and sulfur. Avoiding these foods could lead to nutritional deficiencies. With that, being said please feel free to enjoy goitrogen-containing foods, with the Green Detox recipes, as long as they are permitted on the autoimmune protocol.

RECIPES / INGREDIENTS
1 Granny Smith apple, cored and chopped (organic, unpeeled)
1 ripe kiwi, peeled and chopped
1 cup fresh kale leaves, stems removed
1/2 cup cucumber, peeled and chopped

1/2 cup coconut water
1/2 cup filtered water
1 tablespoon fresh lemon juice
1/2 tablespoon fresh ginger, peeled and grated (optional)
1/2 tablespoon fresh turmeric, peeled and grated (optional)

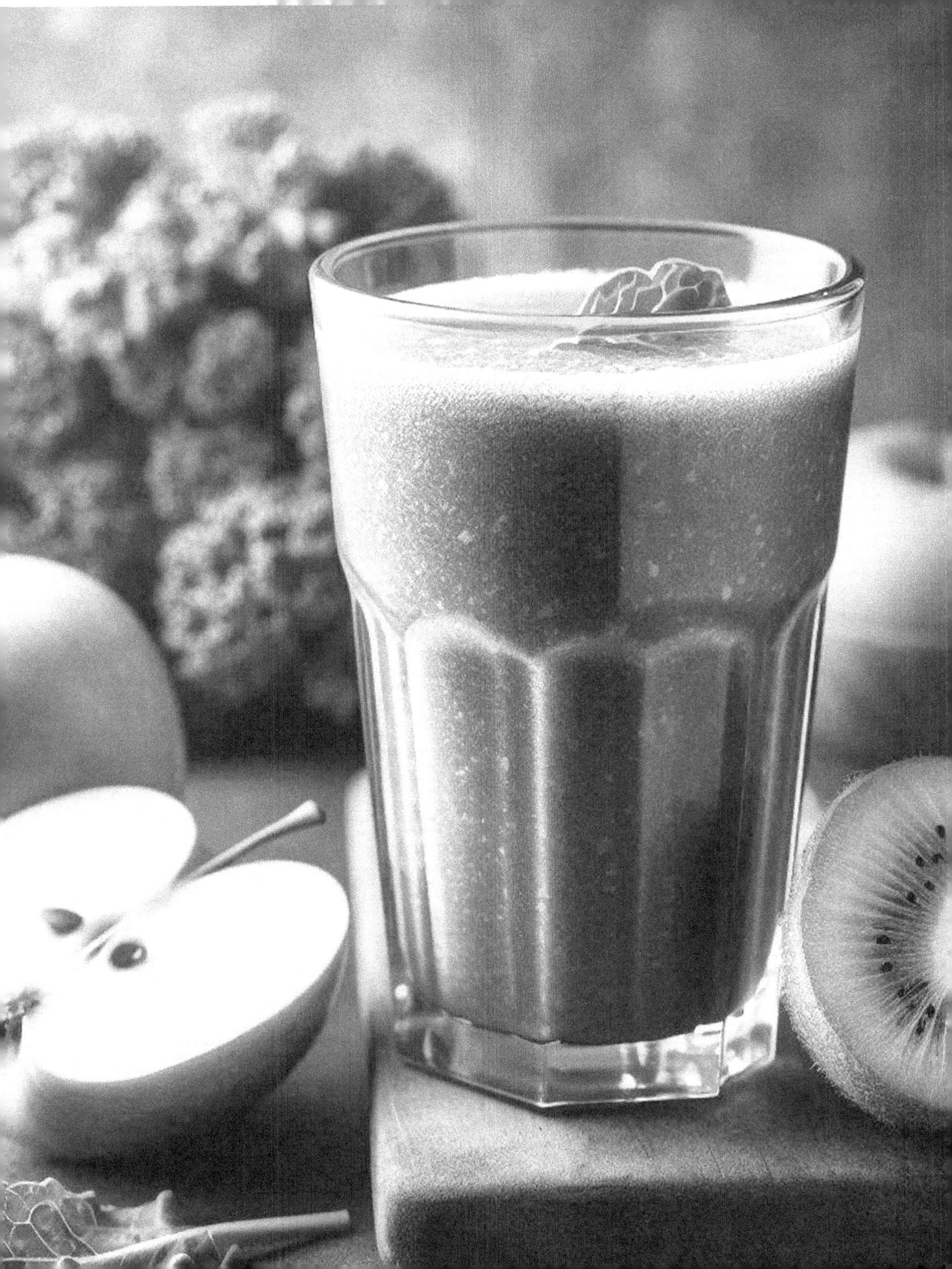

INSTRUCTIONS / DIRECTIONS

Thoroughly wash all fruits and vegetables. If using organic ingredients, you can leave the skin on the apple for added nutrients.

Add the chopped apple, kiwi, kale leaves, cucumber, coconut water, and filtered water to a high-speed blender.

If you like, add the lemon juice, ginger and turmeric for additional flavor and health benefits.

Blend all ingredients until you achieve a smooth consistency.

You may add more coconut water or filtered water if you prefer a thinner consistency

Pour the smoothie into a glass and enjoy immediately for the best taste and nutrient absorption

MORINGA GREEN JUICE

The Moringa tree is often called the "miracle tree" for its remarkable medicinal properties found in nearly every part of the tree, leaves, fruit, sap, oil, roots, bark, seeds, pods, and flowers. This versatile tree, also known as the "drumstick tree," is native to Asia, Africa, and South America and is valued for its widespread use in traditional medicine and nutrition.

This recipe offers numerous health benefits. Moringa leaves contain antioxidants that protect against the harmful effects of free radicals from the environment. Free radicals can contribute to chronic diseases like type 2 diabetes, heart problems, and Alzheimer's. Moringa leaves are particularly rich in vitamin C and beta-carotene, which combat free radicals. They also contain Quercetin, an antioxidant that helps lower blood pressure.

Apart from oats, flaxseeds, and almonds, this juice is a reliable remedy for high cholesterol. High cholesterol is a major factor in heart disease, and drinking this juice has been shown to significantly improve high cholesterol levels. Furthermore, this recipe is packed with essential vitamins such as A, C, B1 (thiamin), B2 (riboflavin), B3 (niacin), B6, and Folate, as well as magnesium, iron, calcium, phosphorus, and zinc.

This juice delivers a potent dose of nutrition with its anti-inflammatory properties. Its antioxidative nature, coupled with its ability to protect cellular health, earns it the title of a new "superfood." It works to reduce the production of inflammatory enzymes and stabilize sugar levels. including this juice into your regular diet can yield numerous health benefits.

This recipe serves as a natural cleanser, helping to detoxify our system. This detoxification process enhances our body's ability to fight off infections, thereby boosting our overall immunity. It helps improve digestion and has mild laxative properties, aiding in the removal of toxins from the body. Which is beneficial for maintaining a healthy gut. There are so many reasons why this juice is my Go-to-rest option.

The vitamins and minerals in Moringa help to support the immune system, and is high in antioxidants, which help combat oxidative stress and may reduce the severity of autoimmune reactions.

RECIPES / INGREDIENTS

1 cup fresh spinach or kale leaves

1/2 cup fresh moringa leaves (or 1 teaspoon moringa powder)

1 cucumber, peeled and chopped

1 green apple, cored and chopped (optional, for sweetness)

1 celery stalk, chopped

1/2 lemon, juiced

1 tablespoon fresh ginger, peeled and chopped

1 cup coconut water(optional)

1/2 cup filtered water (optional, for consistency)

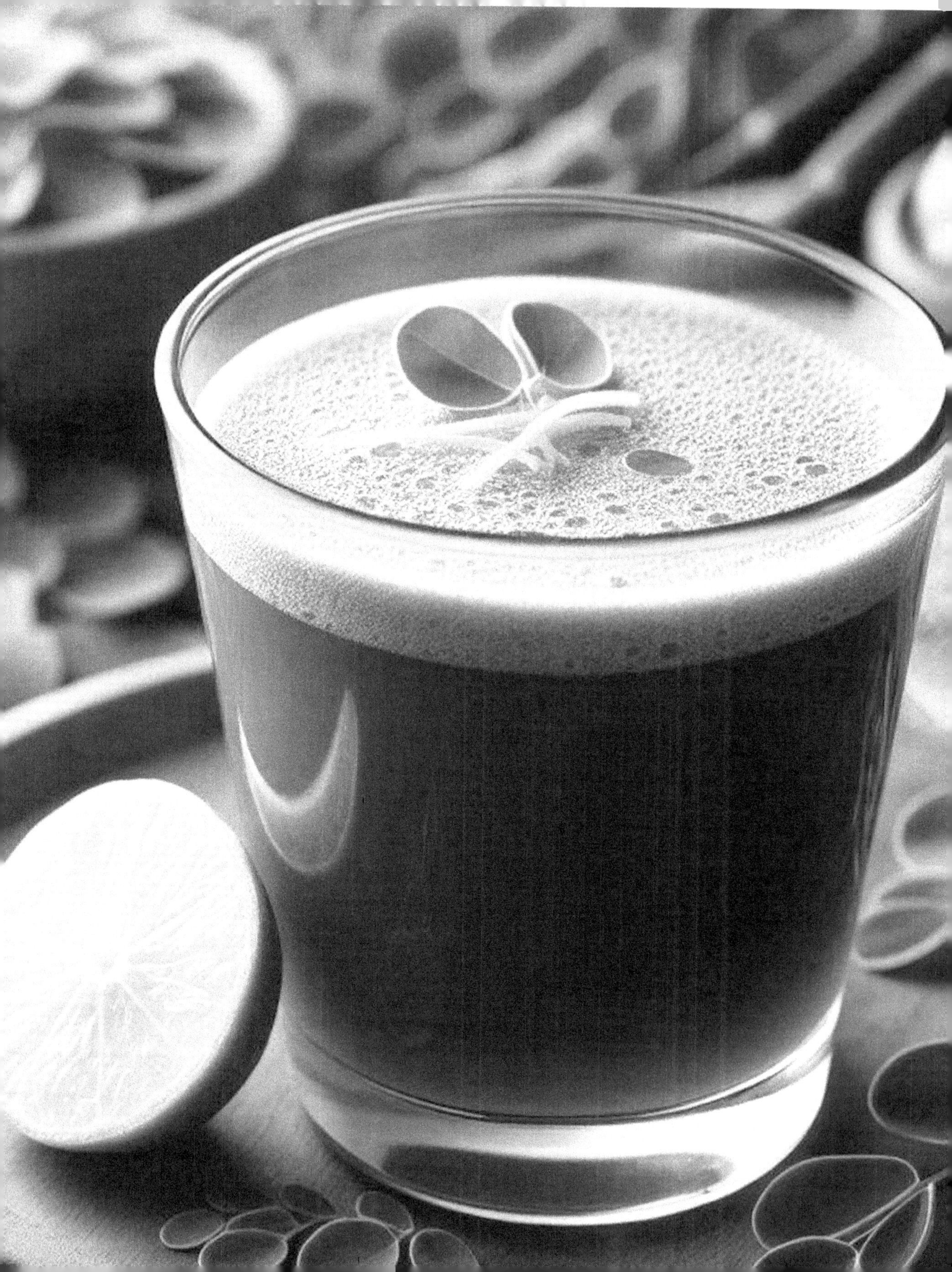

INSTRUCTIONS / DIRECTIONS

Wash all the fresh ingredients thoroughly. If using fresh moringa leaves, remove the stems.

Add spinach or kale, moringa leaves (or powder), cucumber, green apple, celery, lemon juice, ginger, and coconut water into a high-speed blender.

Blend all the ingredients until smooth. Add filtered water if needed to achieve the desired consistency.

Pour the juice into a glass and enjoy immediately for maximum nutrient benefits

PRECAUTIONS

Monitor Your Reaction: *As with any new food, especially on a restrictive diet like AIP, it's essential to introduce moringa gradually and monitor your body's response. Although moringa is generally well-tolerated, but our body reactions can vary.*

Quality of Ingredients: *Ensure you use fresh, high-quality moringa leaves or a reputable brand of moringa powder to avoid contaminants.*

This Green Apple, Carrot, and Orange Juice is not only delicious but also packed with nutrients that support your immune system, Carrots, apples, and oranges make a fantastic trio for boosting our body's defenses and enhancing our immune system. This refreshing juice combines the tartness of green apples, the natural sweetness of carrots, and the zesty burst of oranges.

Green apples and oranges are rich in vitamin C, an essential nutrient that strengthens our immune system and helps our body fight off infections. Vitamin C is also known for its antioxidant properties, which protect our cells from damage. Carrots on the other side are loaded with beta carotene, which our body converts into vitamin A. This vitamin is very important for maintaining a healthy immune system and is known for its role in keeping our skin glowing and healthy.

The combination of apples, carrots, and oranges provides a wide range of antioxidants which reduces inflammation and oxidative stress. The tartness of the green apples perfectly balances the sweetness of the carrots and oranges, creating a delightful flavor that is both refreshing and satisfying. The natural fiber content from the apples and carrots can aid digestion, while oranges provide a good source of calcium and magnesium. Which are both essential minerals for maintaining strong bones, particularly important for seniors to help prevent osteoporosis and other bone-related issues.

RECIPES / INGREDIENTS
2 green apples, cored and chopped
3 medium carrots, peeled and chopped
2 oranges, peeled and segmented

Optional Add-ins for Extra Benefits:

- **Ginger:** Adding a small piece of fresh ginger can enhance the anti-inflammatory properties of the juice and aid in digestion.
- **Turmeric:** A pinch of turmeric can provide additional anti-inflammatory and antioxidant benefits.
- **Spinach:** A handful of spinach can boost the nutrient profile with extra vitamins and minerals without altering the taste significantly.

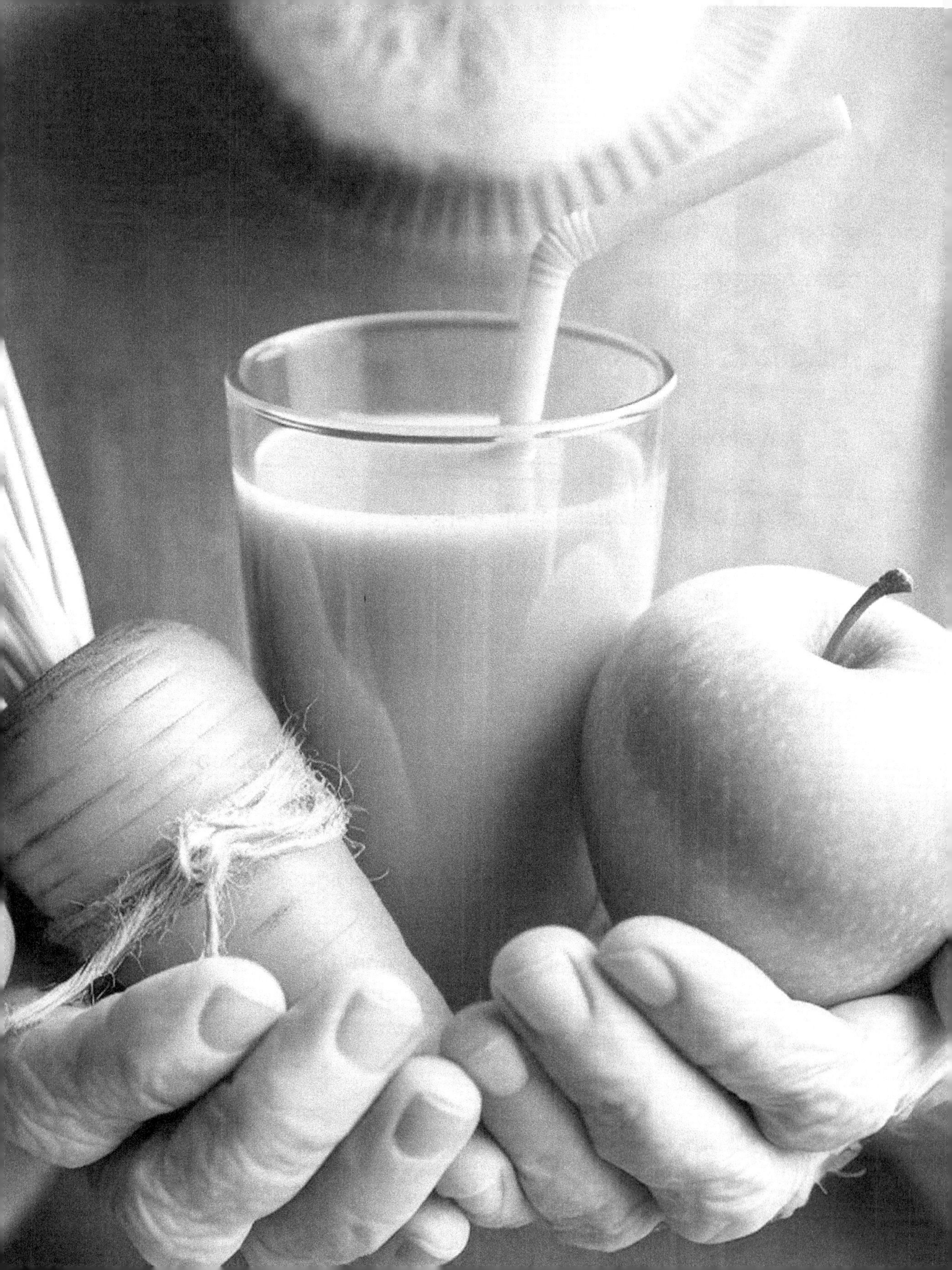

INSTRUCTIONS / DIRECTIONS

Wash all the ingredients thoroughly to remove any dirt and pesticides.

Core the apples and chop them into manageable pieces for your juicer.

Peel and chop the carrots into small pieces.

Peel the oranges and separate them into segments.

Put all the ingredients into your juicer.

Blend until smooth and the juice is well mixed.

TIPS FOR PREPARING THE JUICE:

Organic Produce: Whenever possible, use organic fruits and vegetables to reduce exposure to pesticides and other chemicals, this especially important for seniors and those with sensitive health.

Fresh Ingredients: Use fresh, ripe ingredients to maximize the nutrient content and flavor.

Immediate Consumption: Drink the juice immediately after preparation to take full advantage of its nutritional benefits, as some vitamins can degrade over time when exposed to air.

TROPICAL SUNRISE BLAST

This smoothie combines the delightful and vibrant flavors of pineapple, mango, and banana, evoking a tropical sensation that can transport you to a sunny paradise. The blend of these fruits creates a refreshing and exotic taste experience. Each ingredient in this smoothie adds valuable nutrients. Pineapple and mango are rich in vitamin C, which supports the immune system and overall health. Banana adds potassium and fiber, while unsweetened coconut milk provides healthy fats and a creamy texture.

With the inclusion of coconut milk and juicy fruits, this recipe is hydrating and refreshing, making it perfect for hot days or as a morning pick-me-up, its sweetness is naturally from the ripe fruits, eliminating the need for added sugars or sweeteners. which makes it a wholesome and nutritious option for those seeking a healthier alternative to sugary drinks.

This Tropical Sunrise Smoothie" stands out for its delicious tropical flavors, nutrient density, AIP-friendly composition, natural sweetness, hydrating properties, and versatility. Words will fail me, if I'm to express how I feel, anytime I'm taking a sip from it. It's better to experience it for yourself.

Certain components in pineapple and mango, such as bromelain and other phytochemicals, possess anti-inflammatory properties, these properties Reduces inflammation in the body and also benefit both immune and gut health.

RECIPES / INGREDIENTS
1 cup fresh pineapple chunks
1/2 cup fresh mango chunks
1 small ripe banana
Juice of 1 orange
Juice of 1/2 lemon
1/2-inch piece of fresh ginger, peeled and grated
1 cup unsweetened coconut water or coconut milk (for creamier texture))
Optional: Ice cubes (for extra chill

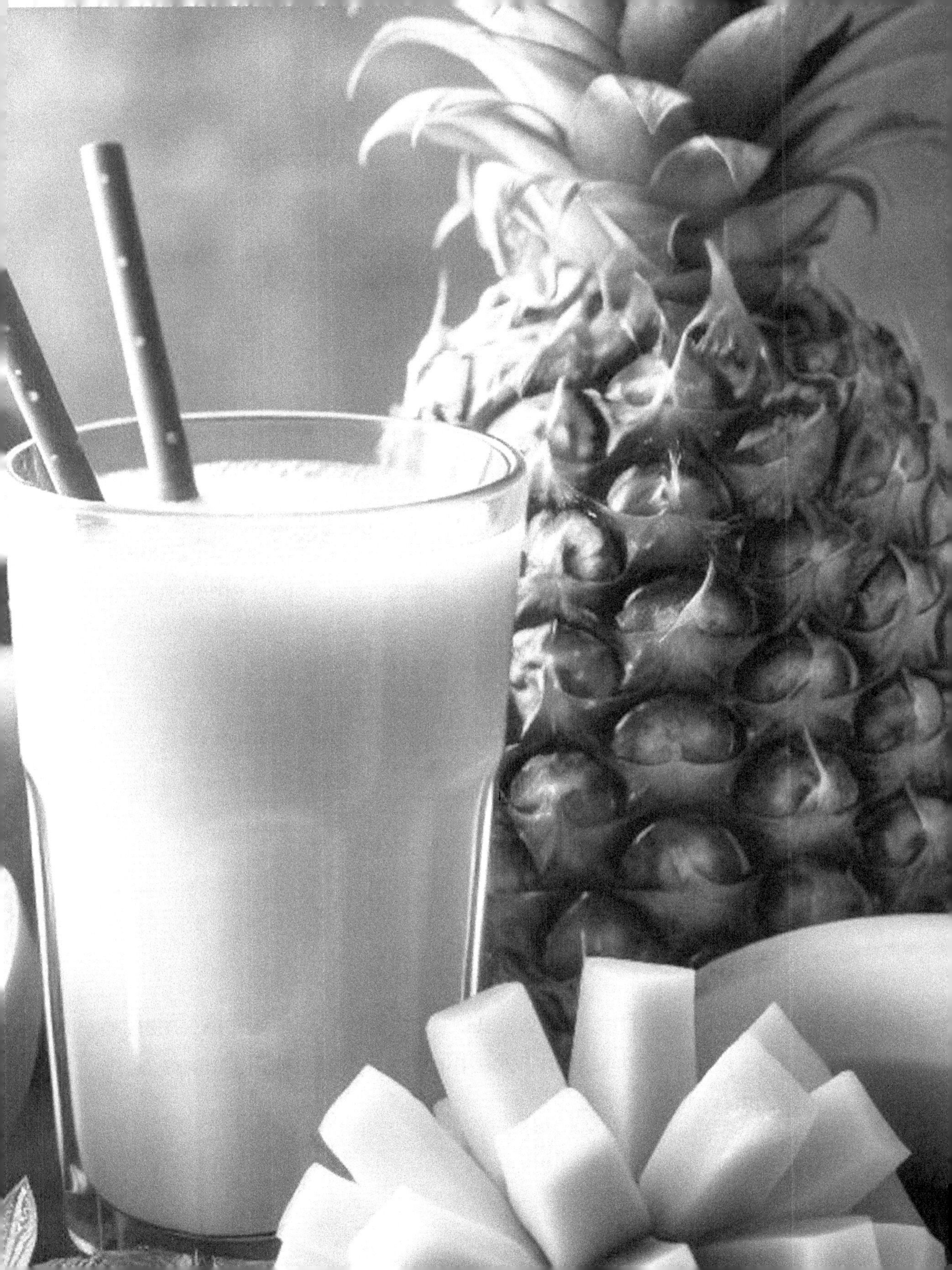

Ensure using whole natural ingredients, without adding sugar or processed ingredients, to get the best nutrients in their most bioavailable form.

INSTRUCTIONS / DIRECTION
Add the pineapple chunks, mango chunks, banana, orange juice, lemon juice, grated ginger, and coconut water (or coconut milk) to a blender.
If desired, add a handful of ice cubes for a colder smoothie.
Blend on high speed until smooth and creamy.
Taste and adjust sweetness by adding more banana or a touch of honey if desired.
Pour into glasses and enjoy immediately

UNIQUE FEATURES

Citrus Burst: The combination of fresh pineapple, mango, orange juice, and lemon juice provide a refreshing citrus burst that's rich in vitamin C.

Ginger Zing: The addition of fresh ginger adds a zesty kick

Coconut Creaminess: Using coconut water or coconut milk adds a creamy texture and provides healthy fats and electrolytes.

Naturally Sweet: The sweetness of ripe fruits like pineapple and banana means no additional sugars are needed.

CUCUMBER, CELERY WITH GREEN APPLE

If you're looking for recipes, for anti-inflammatory diet or juice that support arthritis, then, this delicious and delightful drink is for you. This juice recipes, are rich in anti-inflammatory ingredients, and is ideal, blend to aid in bolstering our body natural defenses and alleviating inflammation.

Fresh juices stand out as some of the finest natural anti-inflammatory beverages. While juicing for inflammation and weight loss enjoys widespread popularity, selecting the correct blend of ingredients is paramount. While anti-inflammatory fruit juices offer health benefits, incorporating vegetables like cucumbers and celery elevates the quality further, as these options typically contain lower sugar content.

Pineapple is undoubtedly one of my preferred anti-inflammatory ingredients, which is why I made sure to include it into this recipe. You may already be familiar with the anti-inflammatory benefits of pineapple and pineapple juice, attributed to its high bromelain content. Ginger is another ingredient that scientific research has demonstrated to have powerful antioxidant and anti-inflammatory properties. It can also aid in reducing muscle pain following intense exercise.

What makes green apple a great addition to this juice recipe? Beyond its delightful flavor, green apple is a rich source of quercetin, a natural antihistamine and anti-inflammatory compound, similar to pineapple. Additionally, low-sugar lemon is included. Studies using animal models have demonstrated that extracts from lemon peel can help reduce inflammation associated with arthritis.

Therefore, when preparing this juice, I highly recommend using the whole lemon, including the peel, for maximum benefits.

If you aim to create an anti-inflammatory smoothie, consider adding some of the fruits and vegetables used in this recipe. Whether you're blending or juicing for health, recipes like this anti-inflammatory juice are essential additions to your routine.

RECIPES / INGRIDENTS

4 stalks of celery
½ cucumber
1 cup of pineapple chunks
½ green apple, cored and chopped
1 cup of spinach leaves
Juice of 1 lemon
1-inch piece of ginger

With a juicer ready, this recipe can be prepared from start to finish in just a few minutes. One serving of this delicious juice provides approximately:

- 114 calories
- 2 grams of protein
- 0 grams of fat
- 28 grams of carbohydrates
- 5.5 grams of fiber
- 16 grams of sugar
- 112 milligrams of sodium

- 81 micrograms of vitamin K (68% DV)
- 1,512 IUs of vitamin A (30% DV)
- 27 milligrams of vitamin C (30% DV)
- 532 milligrams of potassium (11% DV)
- 32 micrograms of folate (8% DV)
- 1.3 milligrams of iron (7.2% DV)
- 66 milligrams of calcium (5.1% DV)
- 12.5 milligrams of magnesium (3% DV)
- 0.2 milligrams of zinc (1.8% DV)

NUTRITION INFORMATION

Calories	114
Sugar	16g
Sodium	112mg
Fat	0g
Carbohydrates	28g
Fiber	5.5g
Protein	2g

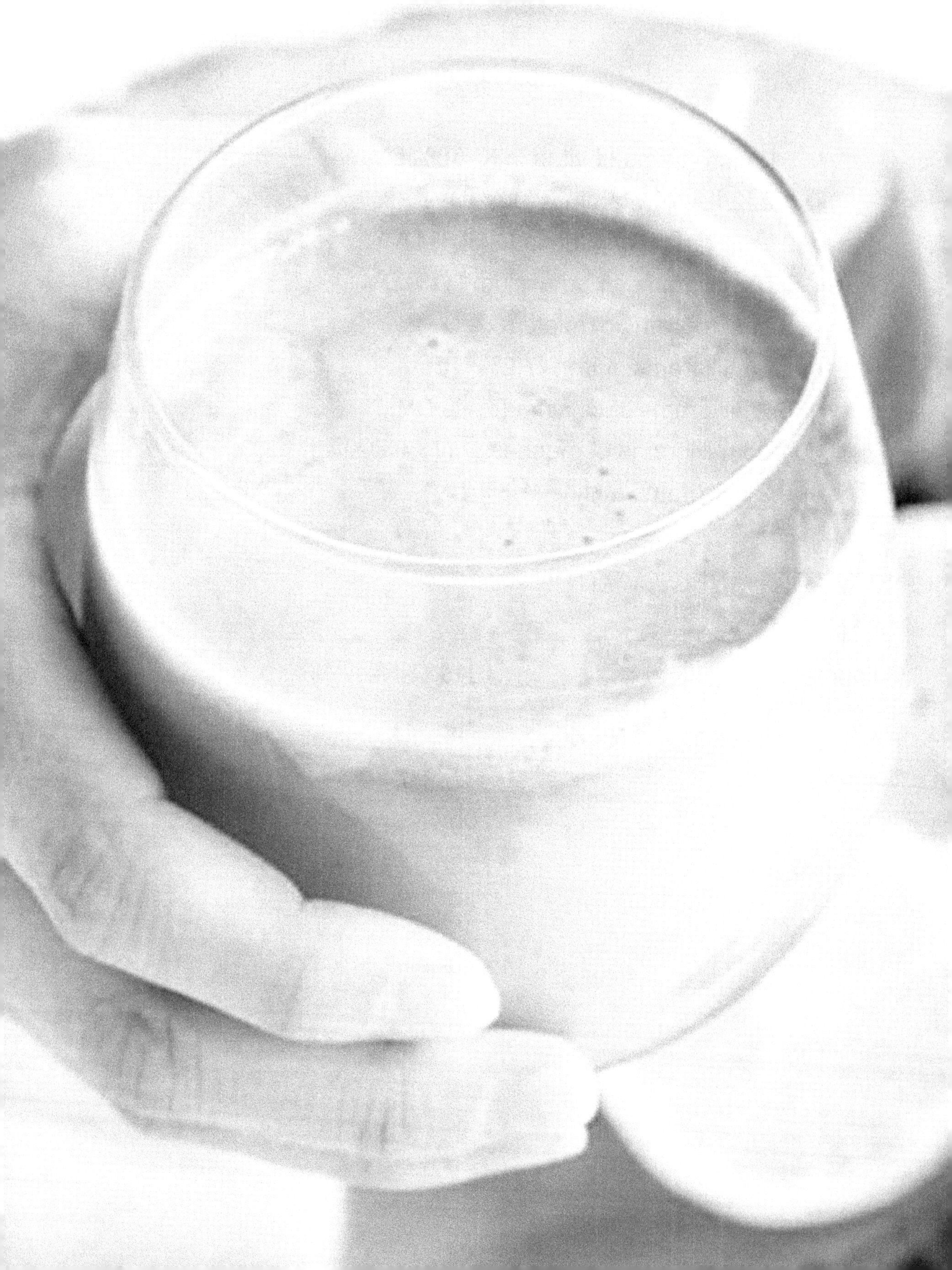

INSTRUCTIONS / DIRECTIONS

Wash the cucumber, celery, lemon, and green apple thoroughly.

Peel the cucumber if desired.

Core and chop the green apple.

Using a juicer, begin by juicing the cucumber and celery stalks.

Next, juice the pineapple chunks and green apple.

Add the juice of one whole lemon to the mixture.

Alternate between juicing the ingredients to ensure even mixing.

Once all ingredients are juiced, stir the mixture well to combine the flavors.

Pour the juice into a glass over ice if desired.

Please note; if you don't have a juicer, you can use your blender. This drink is packed with beneficial nutrients and enzymes.

PAPAYA PASSION REFRESHER

Combining tropical fruits, cucumber, lime, and mint results in a delicious and hydrating juice that not only pleases your palate but also delivers vital nutrients. The Papaya Passion Refresher stands out for its ability to aid digestion, strengthen the immune system, and promote overall wellness.

This juice is one of my favorite because the ingredients in it, such as papaya and cucumber, are known for their digestive benefits. Papaya contains enzymes like papain, which can aid in digestion and help break down proteins. Cucumber is hydrating and gentle on the stomach, making it soothing for those with digestive sensitivities

The combination of tropical fruits and lime in this juice provides a rich source of vitamins and antioxidants that can help strengthen the immune system. Vitamin C from the lime, in particular, supports immune function. The ingredients in this juice have anti-inflammatory properties. Chronic inflammation is a significant issue in autoimmune diseases, and consuming foods with anti-inflammatory properties aid in reducing inflammation and promoting healing.

Beyond its health benefits, this juice is refreshing and delicious, making it an enjoyable and delightful way to include nutrient-dense ingredients in your diet.

RECIPES / INGRIDENTS

1 cup fresh papaya, peeled, seeded, and chopped
1/2 cucumber, peeled and chopped
Juice of 1 lime
A handful of fresh mint leaves
1-2 cups of cold water or coconut water (adjust for desired consistency)
Optional: Ice cubes for serving

When selecting your ingredients, please ensure you choose only the best fresh quality. Tidy up your kitchen or refrigerator and avoid placing them in an unclean and unkept area.

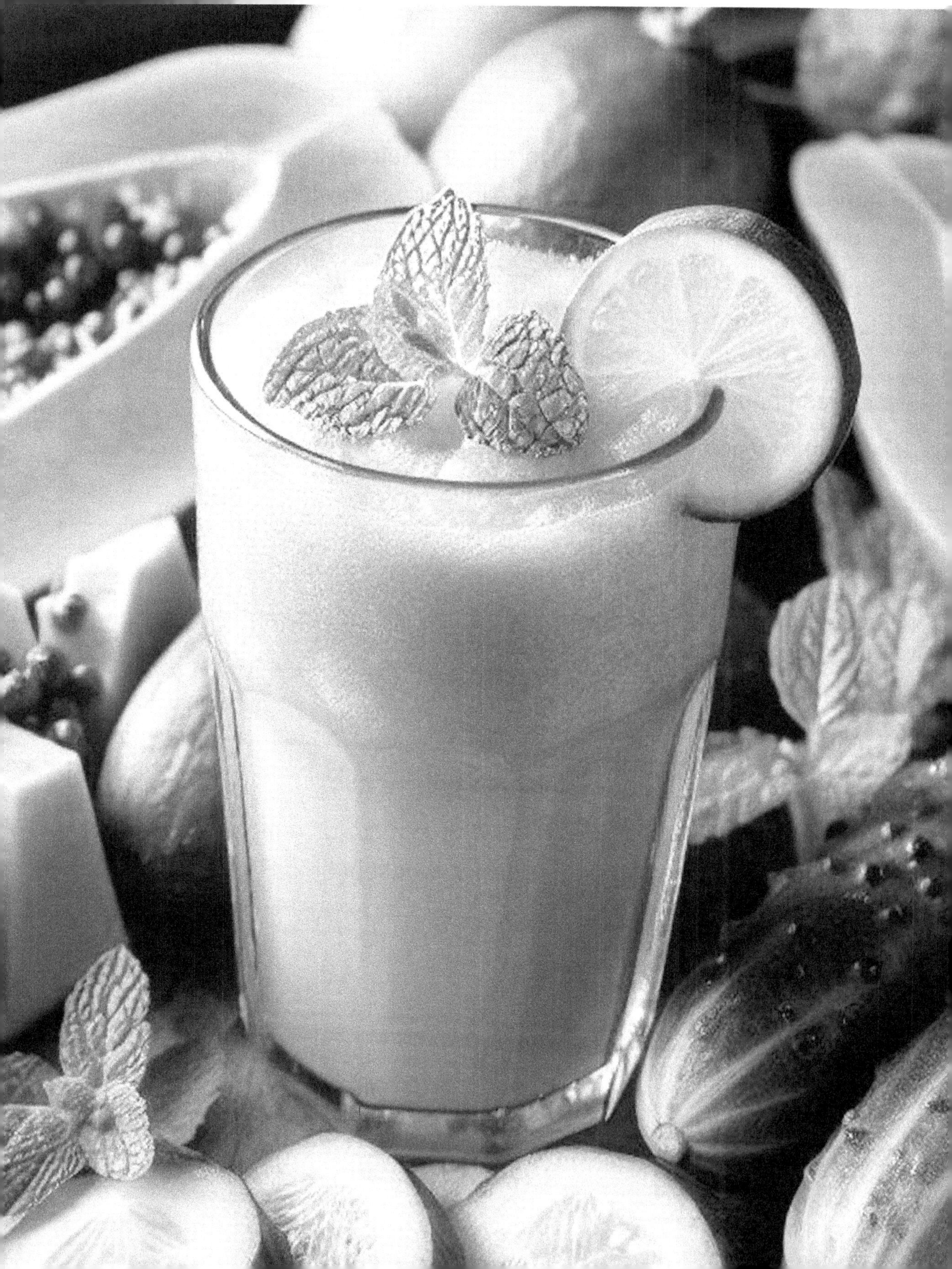

INSTRUCTIONS / DIRECTIONS

In a blender, combine the chopped papaya, cucumber, lime juice, and fresh mint leaves.

Add 1 cup of cold water or coconut water to the blender.

Blend until smooth and well combined. If the mixture is too thick, add more water until you reach your desired consistency.

Taste and adjust by adding more lime juice or mint leaves as needed.

If desired, strain the juice through a fine mesh sieve to remove any pulp.

Pour the juice into glasses filled with ice cubes.

Garnish with a sprig of fresh mint and a slice of lime, if desired.

This juice is not only delicious but also packed with vitamins, minerals, and antioxidants from the papaya, cucumber, lime, and mint. It's a perfect way to stay hydrated, while following the Autoimmune Protocol (AIP). Adjust the ingredients and flavors according to your taste preferences and dietary needs.

PROBIOTIC PINEAPPLE AND BERRY DELIGHT

This blend of ingredients forms a delicious and revitalizing drink while introducing probiotics and other nutrients that support a healthy gut environment. Mixed berries are packed with antioxidants that combat oxidative stress and inflammation in the body. Bananas provide dietary fiber, promoting healthy digestion.

This juice is a nutritious and gut-friendly beverage that can be particularly beneficial for us, especially if you are following the Autoimmune Protocol (AIP). Pineapple contains bromelain, an enzyme that aids in digestion and has anti-inflammatory properties. It is naturally sweet which adds a tropical flavor to the drink. Berries, such as blueberries, strawberries, raspberries, or blackberries, are rich in antioxidants, and they help to combat oxidative stress and also reduces inflammation.

For me, adding Coconut milk or yogurt serves as the base of this drink because they provide healthy fats. Always choose unsweetened varieties to adhere to the AIP guidelines. The inclusion of probiotics in this recipe helps support a healthy gut microbiome, which is essential for anyone with autoimmune conditions. A balanced gut flora can contribute to improved digestion, reduced inflammation, and enhanced immune function. The combination of pineapple, berries, and coconut creates a delicious and refreshing beverage that can be enjoyed as a snack or part of a meal, making it easier to incorporate nutrient-rich foods into your AIP diet.

RECIPES / INGRIDENTS
1 cup fresh pineapple chunks
1 cup mixed berries (blueberries, strawberries, raspberries, or blackberries)
1/2 cup unsweetened coconut milk (canned or homemade)
1/2 cup kefir (probiotic-rich)
1 tablespoon chia seeds

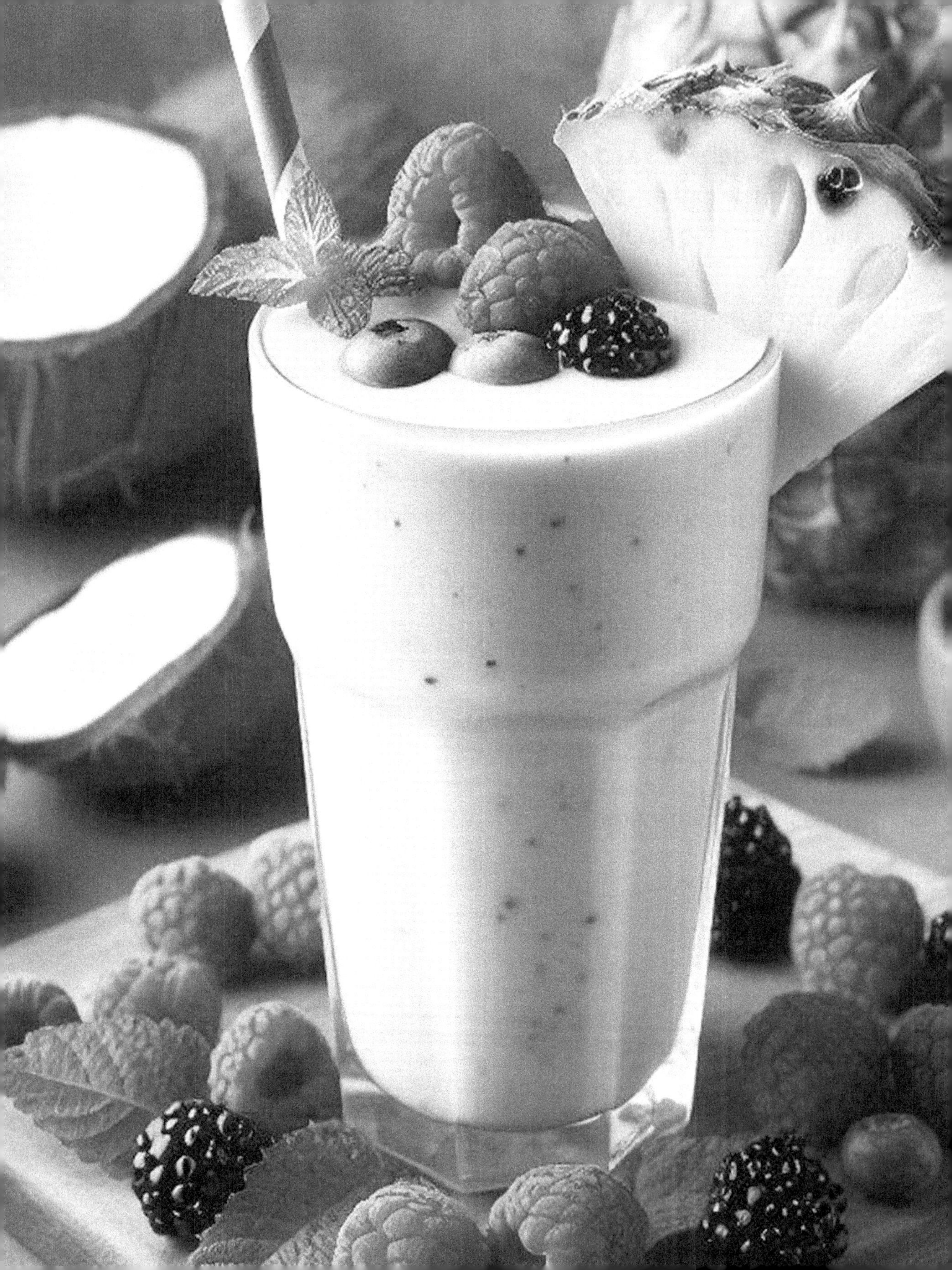

INSTRUCTIONS / DIRECTIONS

In a blender, combine the fresh pineapple chunks and mixed berries.

Add the unsweetened coconut milk and kefir to the blender.

Sprinkle in the chia seeds for added texture and nutrition.

Blend the ingredients until smooth and well combined.

Taste the mixture and adjust sweetness or thickness by adding more coconut milk or kefir if desired.

Pour the probiotic pineapple and berry mixture into glasses.

Optionally, garnish with a few whole berries or a pineapple wedge

This refreshing beverage is packed with probiotics, antioxidants, and omega-3 fatty acids from the chia seeds. Feel free to customize the recipe by using your favorite combination of berries or adjusting the amount of coconut milk and kefir based on your preferred consistency. Ensure that the coconut milk and kefir used are unsweetened and are free of additives.

TIPS FOR AIP-FRIENDLY SATISFACTION

. Use homemade coconut yogurt or AIP-compliant probiotic supplements to ensure the recipe aligns with the AIP guidelines.

. Adjust sweetness based on personal preference and tolerance. You can omit sweeteners altogether or use small amounts of honey or maple syrup if tolerated.

TURMERIC AND CARROT CITRUS ELIXIR

These ingredients combine to form a powerful elixir packed with immune-boosting vitamin C, anti-inflammatory turmeric, and other beneficial compounds. Turmeric, especially, has been extensively studied for its potential health advantages, such as reducing inflammation, promoting joint health, and offering antioxidant benefits.

Turmeric, a key ingredient in this elixir, contains curcumin, a potent anti-inflammatory compound. Curcumin helps reduce inflammation in the body, which is important for managing autoimmune conditions characterized by chronic inflammation. Turmeric, carrots, and citrus fruits (like oranges or lemons) are all rich in antioxidants. Antioxidants help combat oxidative stress and free radicals, which can contribute to inflammation and damage to cells. Taking antioxidant-rich foods supports our health and immune function.

Carrots on the other hand, are a good source of dietary fiber, which supports gut health by promoting regular bowel movements and feeding beneficial gut bacteria. A healthy gut microbiome is important for immune regulation. This Turmeric and Carrot Citrus Elixir is made from natural ingredients without additives or processed sugars. Avoiding processed foods and focusing on nutrient-dense, whole foods supports healing and reduces inflammation.

RECIPES / INGREDIENTS
3 medium carrots, peeled and chopped
2 medium oranges, peeled and segmented
1/2 tablespoon fresh ginger, peeled and grated
1/2 tablespoon fresh turmeric, peeled and grated
Juice of 1/2 small lemon
1 cup filtered water
1 tablespoon honey or maple syrup (optional, omit for strict AIP)

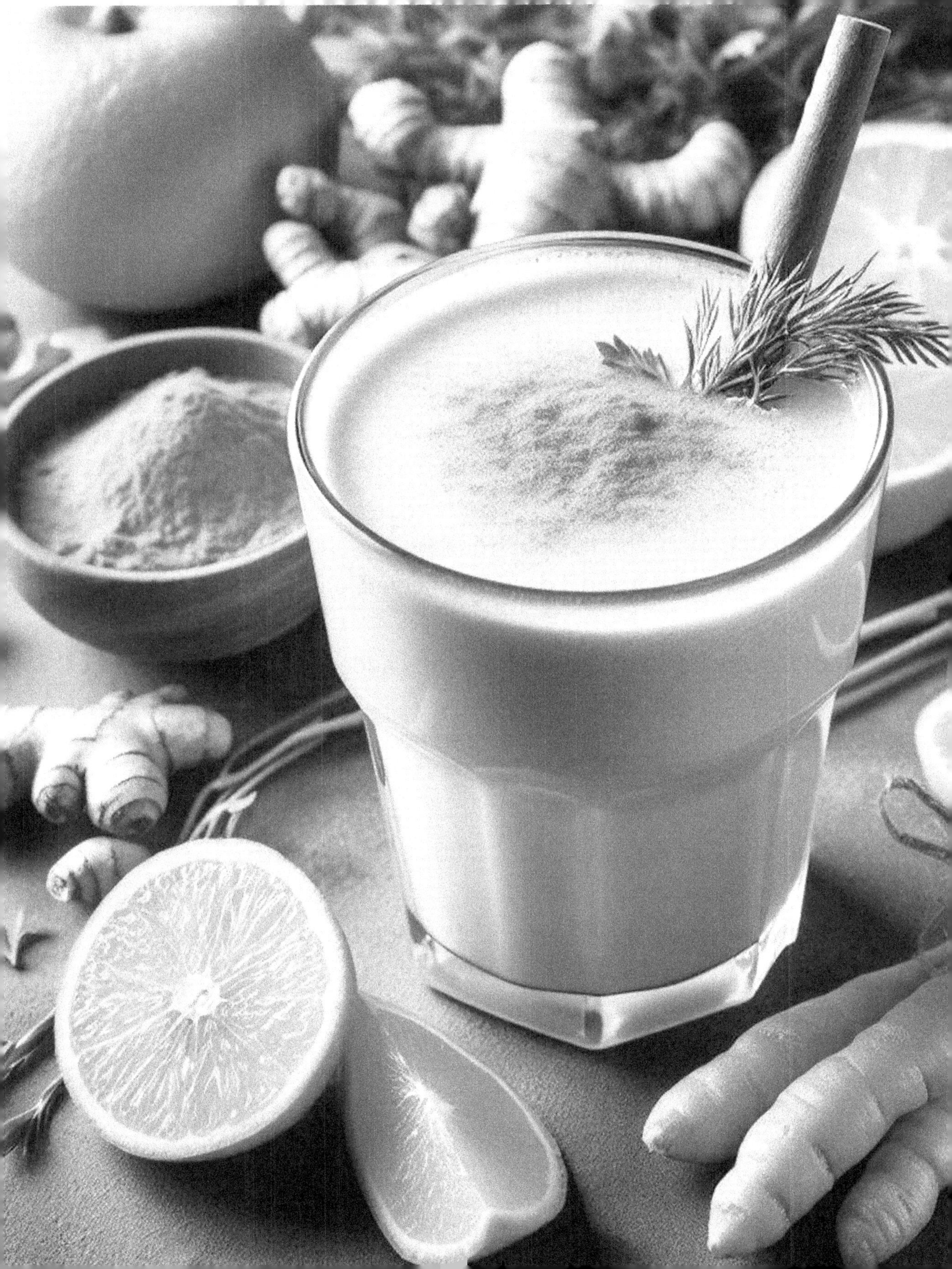

INSTRUCTIONS / DIRECTIONS

In a blender, combine the chopped carrots, orange segments, grated ginger, grated turmeric, and lemon juice.

Add 1 cup of filtered water to the blender.

Blend the ingredients until smooth and well combined.

Taste the elixir and adjust sweetness by adding 1 tablespoon of honey or maple syrup if desired (optional, omit for strict AIP).

Blend again briefly to incorporate any added sweetener.

If the mixture is too thick, you can add more water to reach your desired consistency.

Pour the Turmeric and Carrot Citrus Elixir into glasses.

Optionally, garnish with a slice of orange or a sprig of fresh mint

BEETROOT WITH MINTY MELON SOOTHER

The Beetroot with Minty Melon Soothe brings a range of health benefits to the table. Watermelon, a key ingredient, is not only hydrating but also rich in vitamins A and C, as well as antioxidants like lycopene, which helps to protect against oxidative stress and inflammation. Cucumber, another essential component, adds to the hydration factor and contributes to our overall digestive health due to its fiber content, aiding in regular bowel movements and supporting gut health.

Mint leaves are well-known for their soothing properties, which calms the digestive system and alleviate discomfort. Lime, if included, provides an additional burst of vitamin C, supporting the immune system and promoting collagen production for healthy skin and tissues. Aloe vera gel, known for its potential anti-inflammatory and digestive benefits, can further enhance the overall wellness impact of this juice.

These ingredients create a well-rounded juice that not only supports hydration and digestion but also delivers a dose of essential nutrients crucial for overall health and well-being. The combination of antioxidants, vitamins, fiber, and soothing properties makes the Beetroot with Minty Melon Soothe a refreshing and nutritious addition to your diet.

Aloe vera gel does not need to be added to this Beetroot with Minty Melon Soothe if you prefer not to include it. Aloe vera is optional and can be omitted based on personal preference or dietary considerations.

RECIPES / INGREDIENTS
1 small beetroot, peeled and chopped
2 cups cubed watermelon (seedless)
1/2 cucumber, peeled and chopped
Handful of fresh mint leaves
Juice of 1 lime
1-2 cups filtered water (adjust for desired consistency)

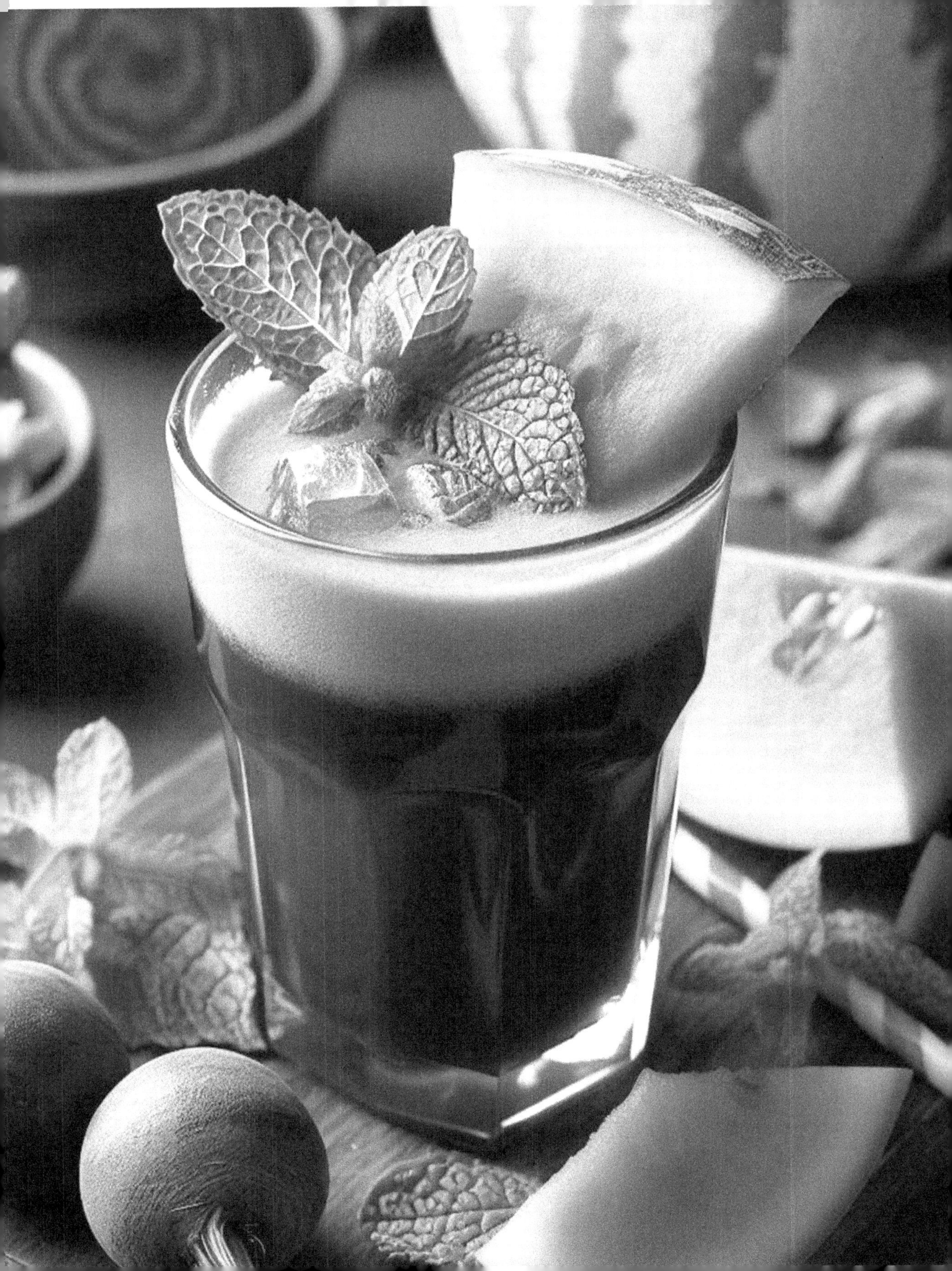

INSTRUCTIONS / DIRECTIONS

Prepare the ingredients by washing, peeling (if necessary), and chopping the beetroot, watermelon, cucumber, and mint leaves.

Place the chopped beetroot, watermelon, cucumber, and mint leaves into a blender.

Squeeze the juice of one lime into the blender.

Add 1-2 cups of filtered water, depending on how thick or thin you prefer your juice.

Blend on high speed until smooth and well combined.

Taste the juice and adjust the sweetness and tanginess by adding more lime juice or watermelon if desired.

Pour the Beetroot with Minty Melon Soothe into glasses.

Optionally, garnish with a mint leaf or slice of cucumber for decoration.

Serve chilled and enjoy this refreshing and nutrient-packed beverage

WATERMELON MINT

Watermelon is the perfect summer delight! Despite its sweet and refreshing nature, watermelon is a nutritional powerhouse. Not only is it relatively low in sugar compared to other fruits, but it is also packed with vitamin C. Watermelon also contains antioxidants and anti-inflammatory compounds, along with potassium and magnesium. Its high-water content makes it an excellent post-workout snack.

I absolutely love watermelon! With the availability of smaller and seedless varieties, there's no excuse not to enjoy it. Mint enhances watermelon's fresh taste, making them a perfect pair for smoothies, juices, and teas.

You can cut up the watermelon and freeze it ahead of time, but if you're like me, who doesn't always plan ahead, you can blend your smoothie with about half a cup of crushed ice. Don't worry about the watermelon seeds; they'll blend right in with the other ingredients. The seeds are packed with nutrients, just like flax and chia seeds.

I like to add protein to my smoothies. plain protein flavor works well with this recipe. It might seem unusual to add milk to watermelon, but trust me, it gives the smoothie a nice creamy texture. Any type of milk will work, but coconut milk is especially tasty in this smoothie.

For an extra anti-inflammatory boost, I like to add maca powder and beet root powder. However, these are not essential ingredients and can be omitted if you prefer. But the key thing I want you to note are these functions of the recipes I mentioned.

- Watermelon is rich in vitamins A and C; watermelon supports immune function and skin health. Its high-water content also helps to keep us hydrated, which is crucial for maintaining overall health.

- Mint contains anti-inflammatory properties that can help soothe the digestive tract and support immune health.

- Maca Powder is known for its adaptogenic properties, maca can help balance hormones and improve overall energy, which supports a healthy immune system.

- Beet Root Powder are high in antioxidants and nitrates, beet root powder can improve blood flow and reduce inflammation, supporting cardiovascular and immune health.
- Protein Powder helps to repair and build tissues, which is essential for maintaining a strong immune system.

- Coconut Milk contains lauric acid, which has antimicrobial properties that can help fight infections.

2 cups fresh watermelon chunks (seeds can be left in for extra nutrients)

1/2 cup fresh mint leaves

1/2 cup crushed ice

1/2 cup coconut milk (unsweetened)

1 scoop plain protein powder (optional)

1 teaspoon maca powder (optional)

1 teaspoon beet root powder (optional)

This smoothie is a delicious and nutritious way to start your day, providing hydration, essential nutrients, and immune-boosting benefits in one refreshing drink.

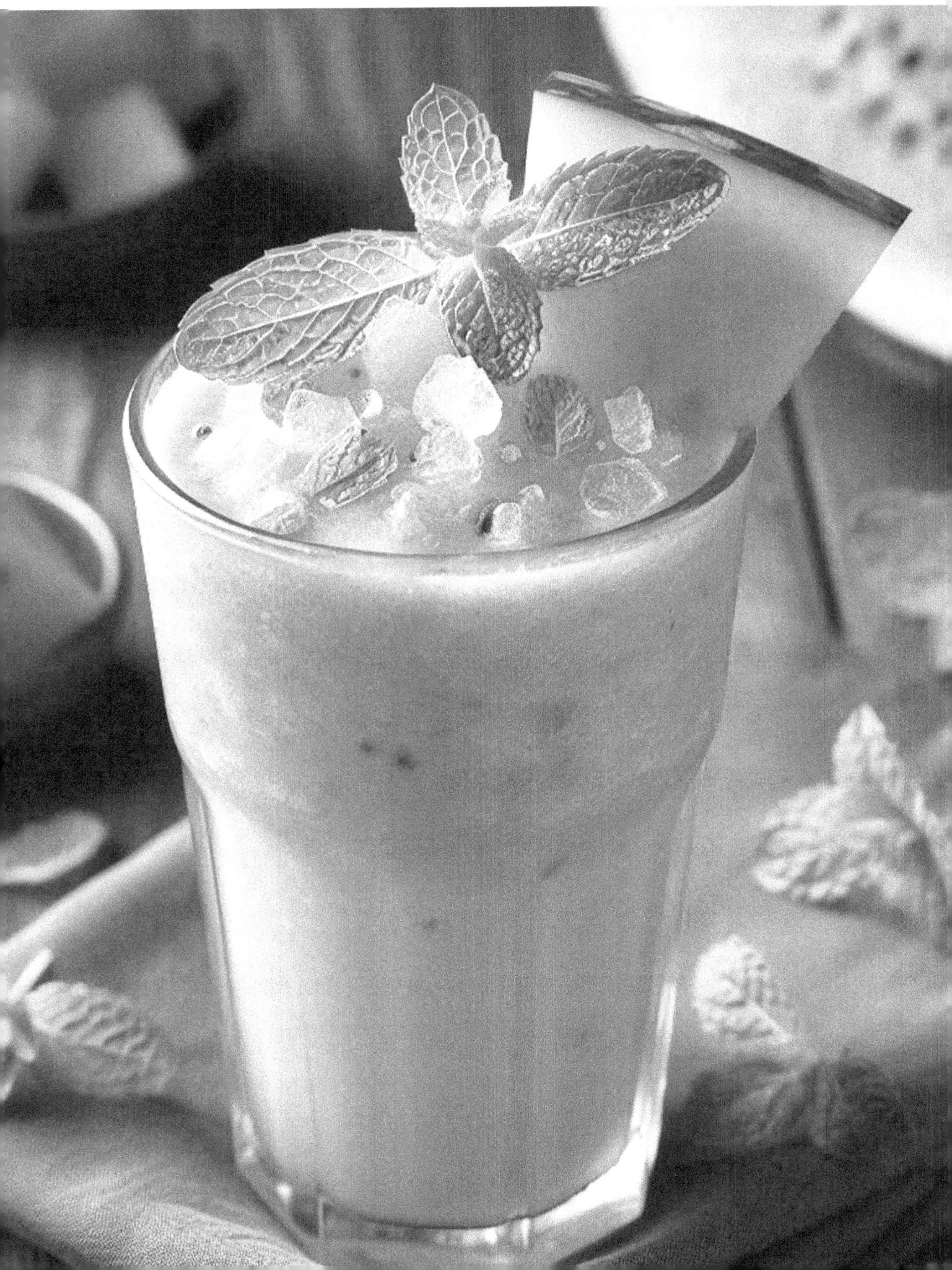

INSTRUCTIONS / DIRECTIONS

Wash and chunk the watermelon. Rinse the mint leaves thoroughly.

Add the watermelon chunks, fresh mint leaves, crushed ice, and coconut milk to the blender.

Add the protein powder, maca powder, and beet root powder to the blender.

Blend all ingredients until you achieve a smooth and creamy consistency. If needed, add more coconut milk or water to reach your desired thickness.

Pour the smoothie into a glass and enjoy immediately

Golden milk, also known as turmeric milk or "haldi doodh" in India, is a traditional beverage known for its health benefits. The primary ingredients typically include milk (dairy or plant-based), turmeric, black pepper, and often other spices and sweeteners. Golden milk is the ultimate healthy, healing, and anti-inflammatory drink.

I like to drink this immediately after blending, but I also enjoy pouring some into a flask to take on a day trip. There's nothing better than having a brisk walk and then enjoying a cup of piping hot golden milk when I return to the car. I first learned about golden milk during my travels in India and was amazed by how simple yet healing this drink is.

To enhance this recipe, I recommend adding orange and dates for extra richness and flavor. This Golden Milk with Orange and Dates is super tasty and very good for us. It's full of healthy nutrients that helps our body stay strong, especially if you have any health problems. The mix of turmeric, ginger, and cinnamon, along with the orange and dates, makes it great for fighting inflammation and boosting the immune system. Plus, it improves our digestive health and nutrient absorption. So let take a quick view at the amazing benefits of this recipes and why it should be among the top ten recipes on the table;

1. Anti-Inflammatory Properties:

Turmeric: Contains curcumin, a powerful anti-inflammatory compound that can help reduce chronic inflammation associated with autoimmune conditions.

Ginger and Cinnamon: Both spices are known for their anti-inflammatory and antioxidant properties, which further aid in reducing inflammation.

2. Digestive Health:

Ginger: Known for its digestive benefits, ginger helps soothe the digestive tract and reduces symptoms like nausea and indigestion.

Dates: High in fiber, and also helps in improving digestion and support gut health.

3. Immune Support:

Orange Juice: Rich in vitamin C, which is essential for a healthy immune system. Vitamin C helps to protect the body against infections and also support our immune function.

Cinnamon: Contains antibacterial and antiviral properties that can help fight infections.

4. Nutrient-Rich:

Coconut Milk: Provides healthy fats and is a good source of vitamins and minerals, including magnesium, which is important for muscle and nerve function.

Dates: Besides fiber, dates are a good source of several vitamins and minerals, including potassium, magnesium, and vitamin B6.

5. Enhanced Absorption:

Black Pepper: The piperine in black pepper enhances the absorption of curcumin from turmeric, making the anti-inflammatory benefits of turmeric more effective.

6. Natural Sweetness:

Maple Syrup and Dates: Offer a natural sweetness without the need for refined sugars, making this drink suitable for every senior and those following the AIP diet.

Like I said earlier, don't let aging stop you from enjoying the things you love. It's a blessing and a privilege to experience life to the fullest, and making this Golden Milk with Orange and Dates is a great way to support your health and keep doing what you enjoy.

2 cups coconut milk (or any AIP-approved milk)

1 teaspoon ground turmeric

1 teaspoon ground cinnamon

1/2 teaspoon ground ginger

1/4 teaspoon black pepper (to enhance turmeric absorption)

2 tablespoons pure maple syrup (optional, for sweetness)

1 orange, juiced

2-3 Medjool dates, pitted

1/2 teaspoon vanilla extract (optional)

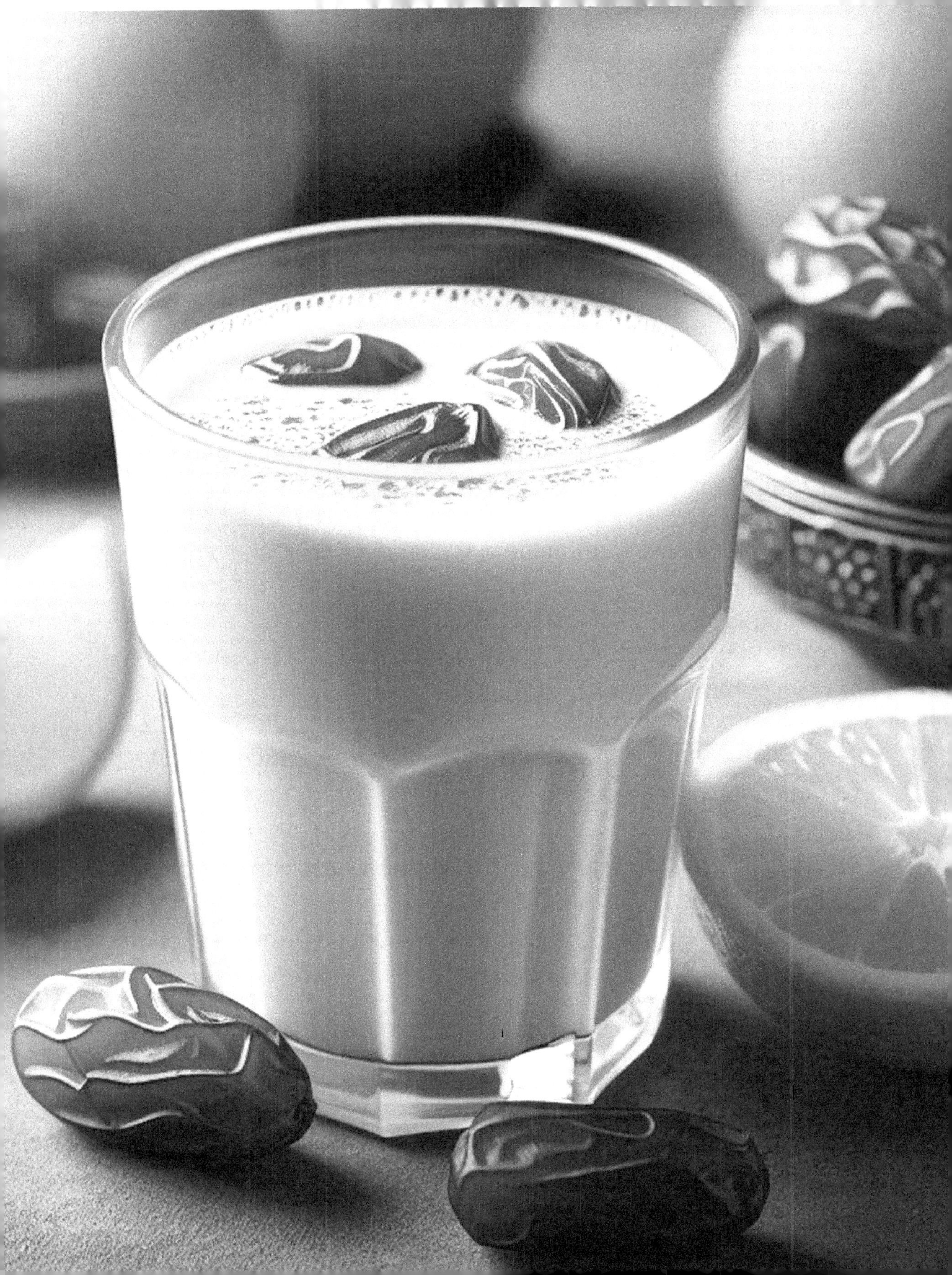

INSTRUCTIONS / DIRECTIONS

Pit the dates and soak them in warm water for about 10 minutes to soften.

Juice the orange and set aside.

In a blender, combine the soaked dates and orange juice. Blend until smooth.

In a small saucepan, pour in the coconut milk and warm over medium heat.

Add the turmeric, cinnamon, ginger, and black pepper to the warm milk. Stir well to combine.

Add the date and orange mixture to the saucepan. Stir to combine all ingredients.

Add the maple syrup if using and vanilla extract for extra flavor.

Simmer the mixture on low heat for about 5-7 minutes, stirring occasionally. Do not let it boil.

Once the mixture is well combined and heated through, remove from heat.

Pour the golden milk into mugs and enjoy immediately for the best flavor and benefits

For this recipe, you can use both fresh and dry ingredients reasons, because using a combination of fresh and dry ingredients allows flexibility in preparation while ensuring you still get the health benefits %100

AUTOIMMUNE COMPLIANT SMOOTHIE

The Autoimmune Protocol (AIP) diet focuses on reducing inflammation, supporting gut health, and minimizing autoimmune responses. With the right ingredients, you can create delicious and nutritious smoothies that align with AIP guidelines. One such creation is the Autoimmune Compliant Smoothie, which combines a range of health-boosting ingredients that focuses on individuals following the AIP diet.

I was inspired to create this particular recipe during a recent trip to Europe. Specifically, I was in Paris, walking along a bustling street in the early afternoon. Feeling low on energy after missing lunch, I was eagerly searching for a healthy option (adhering to the Autoimmune Protocol while traveling can be challenging). I soon spotted a food stall ahead that was selling freshly squeezed juices. Intrigued and thirsty, I ordered a green juice and observed as the vendor expertly combined various fresh ingredients.

The resulting juice was extraordinary, bursting with vibrant flavors and raw goodness, leaving a lasting impression on me. I recreated the recipe today with a few modifications for my personal enjoyment! If you're not a fan of kale, feel free to substitute it with another leafy green, such as chard or even arugula.

RECIPES / INGREDIENTS
1 medium green apple (Granny Smith), seeded
1/2 cucumber, peeled (approx. 1 cup or 145 g or 5 oz)
Juice of 1/2 lime
Juice of 1/2 lemon
1 TBSP fresh ginger, chopped (approx. 7 - 8 g)
1 cup kale, chopped and packed (approx. 18 g or 7 oz)
1 cup coconut water
1 TBSP unflavored gelatin powder (optional)

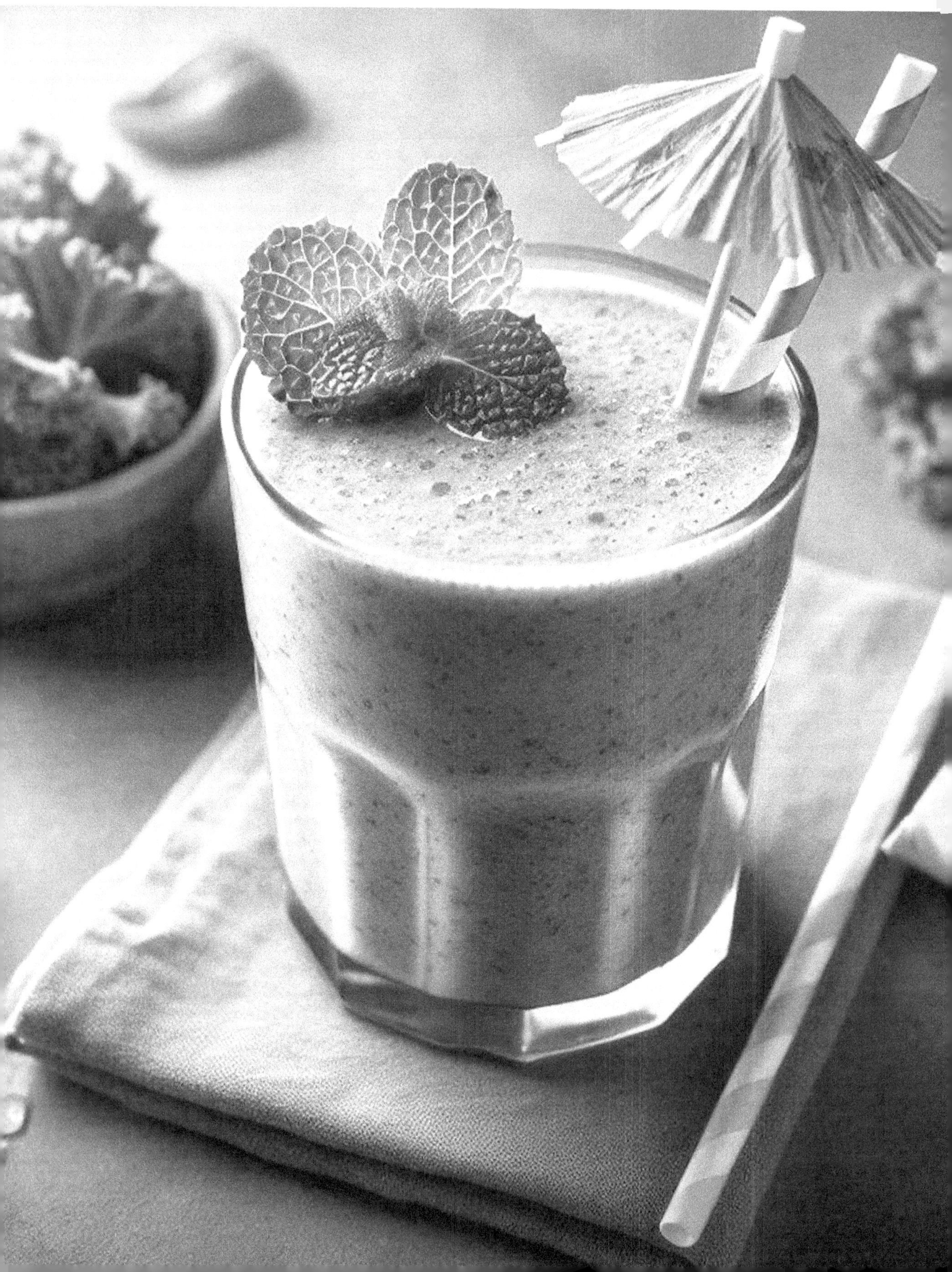

INSTRUCTIONS / DIRECTIONS

First, wash and chop your green apple, cucumber, ginger, and kale. Make sure you remove all the seeds from the apple.

Toss the chopped apple, cucumber, lime juice, lemon juice, fresh ginger, and kale into your blender.

Pour in the coconut water to help everything blend smoothly.

If you want an extra boost, add a tablespoon of unflavored gelatin powder. It's great for your gut.

Blend it all up until you get a nice and smooth texture.

Pour your smoothie into a glass and drink it right away for the best taste and benefits.

This Autoimmune Compliant Smoothie. is packed with ingredients that are perfect for supporting your health and well-being. Ginger, kale, cucumbers, lime, lemon, green apple, and coconut water are all fantastic ingredients, but I'd like to draw your attention specifically to kale. Kale is exceptional because it helps cleanse the liver and supports the body's natural detox processes, which is very important in our general health.

VEGGIE CLEANSE

Spring is a time for renewal, both inside and out. During winter, we often overeat during the holidays, gain weight, and become more sedentary. But spring invites us to start moving again. We pack away winter gear, clean our homes, and prepare our gardens for the warmer weather ahead. Our bodies can also benefit from this seasonal renewal with a Veggie Cleanse Smoothie. Cleansing not only helps shake off the winter blues but also offers a wide range of health benefits, according to research.

Our body naturally cleanses itself every day through its eliminative systems, which expel waste via stool, urine, sweat, and exhaled breath. The liver, a major detoxifying organ, releases its end products through these same channels. The body constantly works to eliminate unnecessary or harmful substances, which can include indigestible fiber, food additives, pesticides, and other pollutants. By intentionally drinking this Veggie Cleanse Smoothie, we actively support and enhance our body's natural cleansing processes.

This smoothie helps in supporting and enhancing the body's natural cleansing processes by providing essential nutrients that our body needs. To be exact, spinach is loaded with chlorophyll, which helps to detoxify the liver and improve digestion. It is also high in fiber, which supports healthy bowel movements and the elimination of toxins through the digestive system. The vitamins and minerals in spinach, such as vitamins A, C, and K, supports our overall immune function and cellular health.

RECIPES / INGREDIENTS
1 cup spinach leaves (rich in vitamins A, C, and K, as well as iron and magnesium)
1 cucumber, peeled and chopped (hydrating and contains antioxidants)
2 celery stalks, chopped (anti-inflammatory and supports digestion)
1 green apple, cored and chopped (provides quercetin, a natural antihistamine and anti-inflammatory compound)
1/2 cup pineapple chunks (contains bromelain, which aids digestion and reduces inflammation)

| Juice of 1 lemon (rich in vitamin C and supports detoxification) |
| 1 cup coconut water (hydrating and rich in electrolytes) |
| 1-inch piece of fresh ginger, peeled (anti-inflammatory and supports digestion) |

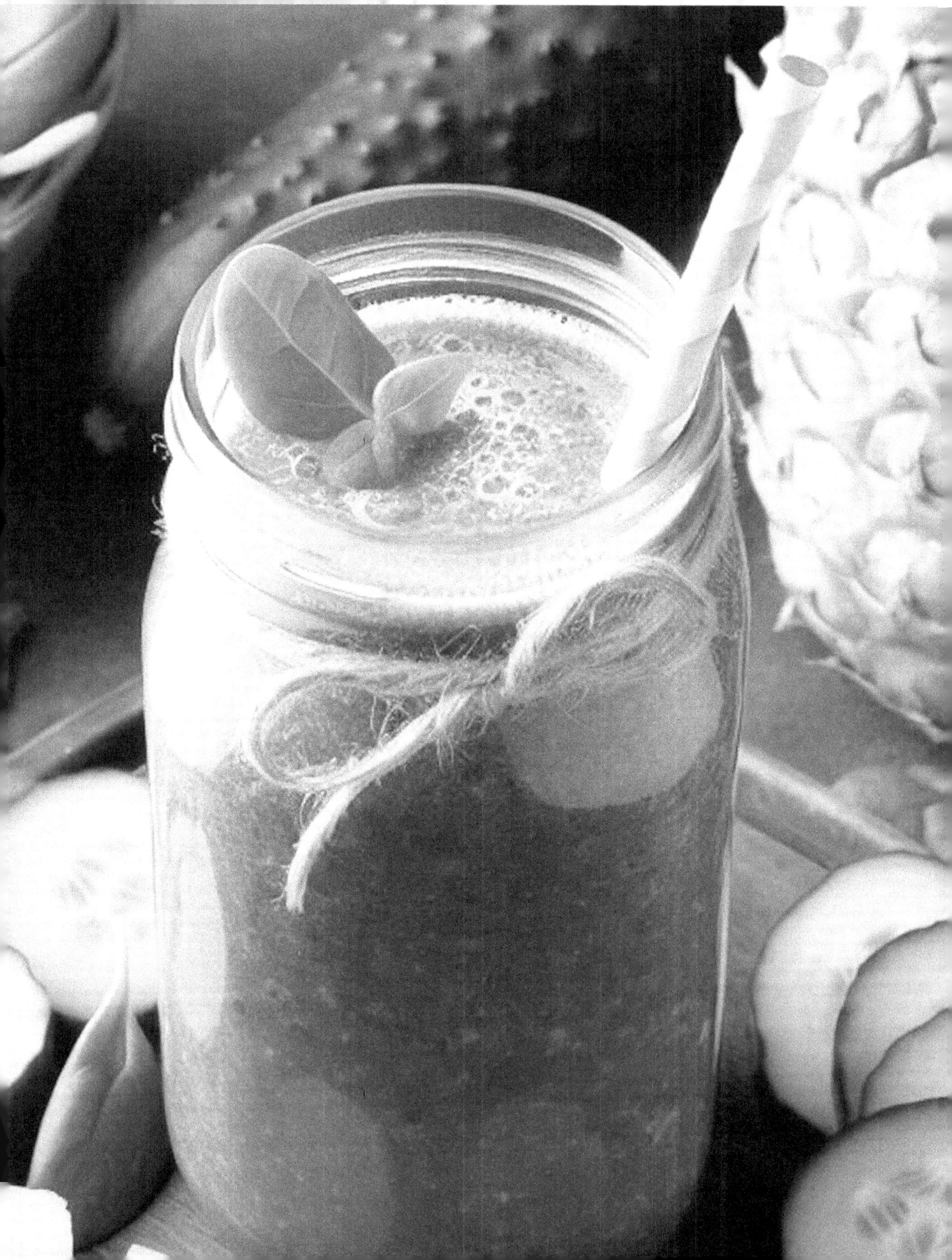

INSTRUCTIONS / DIRECTIONS

Wash all the vegetables and fruits thoroughly.

Peel and chop the cucumber.

Chop the celery stalks and green apple.

Peel the fresh ginger.

Juice the lemon.

Add the spinach leaves, cucumber, celery, green apple, pineapple chunks, lemon juice, fresh ginger, and coconut water to a high-speed blender.

Blend on high until smooth and well combined.

Pour the smoothie into a glass and enjoy immediately for maximum freshness and nutrient retention.

PEACHY GINGER SMOOTHIE

The Peachy Ginger Smoothie is a delightful and nutritious option that combines the sweet, juicy flavor of peaches with the zesty kick of fresh ginger.

Why This Smoothie is Ideal for Seniors

- The Peachy Ginger Smoothie is gentle on the digestive system, making it suitable for those who may have sensitive stomachs.
- This smoothie provides a wide range of essential vitamins and minerals that support overall health and well-being.
- The high-water content in peaches and the hydration provided by coconut milk help keep seniors well-hydrated.
- The combination of sweet peaches and spicy ginger makes for a deliciously refreshing drink that seniors will love.

Health Benefits of this Peachy Ginger Smoothie

Anti-Inflammatory Properties

Ginger: *Fresh ginger is well-known for its powerful anti-inflammatory and antioxidant effects and its ability to reduce inflammation and pain associated with conditions like arthritis.*

Ginger aids in digestion by stimulating the production of digestive enzymes, reducing nausea, and improving overall gut health

Peaches: *Peaches are rich in antioxidants like vitamin C and polyphenols, they help to combat oxidative stress and inflammation in the body. It helps in the production of white blood cells and enhances the body's ability to fight infections.*

Coconut Milk: *Unsweetened coconut milk provides healthy fats that support the digestive system and help with the absorption of fat-soluble vitamins. Coconut milk is also hydrating, it provides essential minerals like potassium, magnesium, and calcium, which are important for maintaining healthy blood pressure and bone health in seniors.*

Honey (optional): *Honey adds a touch of natural sweetness without causing a spike in blood sugar levels. It also has antibacterial properties and can soothe a sore throat.*

RECIPE / INGREDIENTS

1 cup frozen peaches
1 tablespoon fresh ginger, chopped
1 cup unsweetened coconut milk
1 tablespoon honey (optional)

Ensure the peaches are ripe and the ginger is fresh to maximize the nutritional benefits and flavor. If possible, choose organic peaches and ginger to reduce exposure to pesticides and chemicals. Adjust the amount of honey or omit it if you prefer a less sweet smoothie, particularly if you are monitoring your sugar intake.

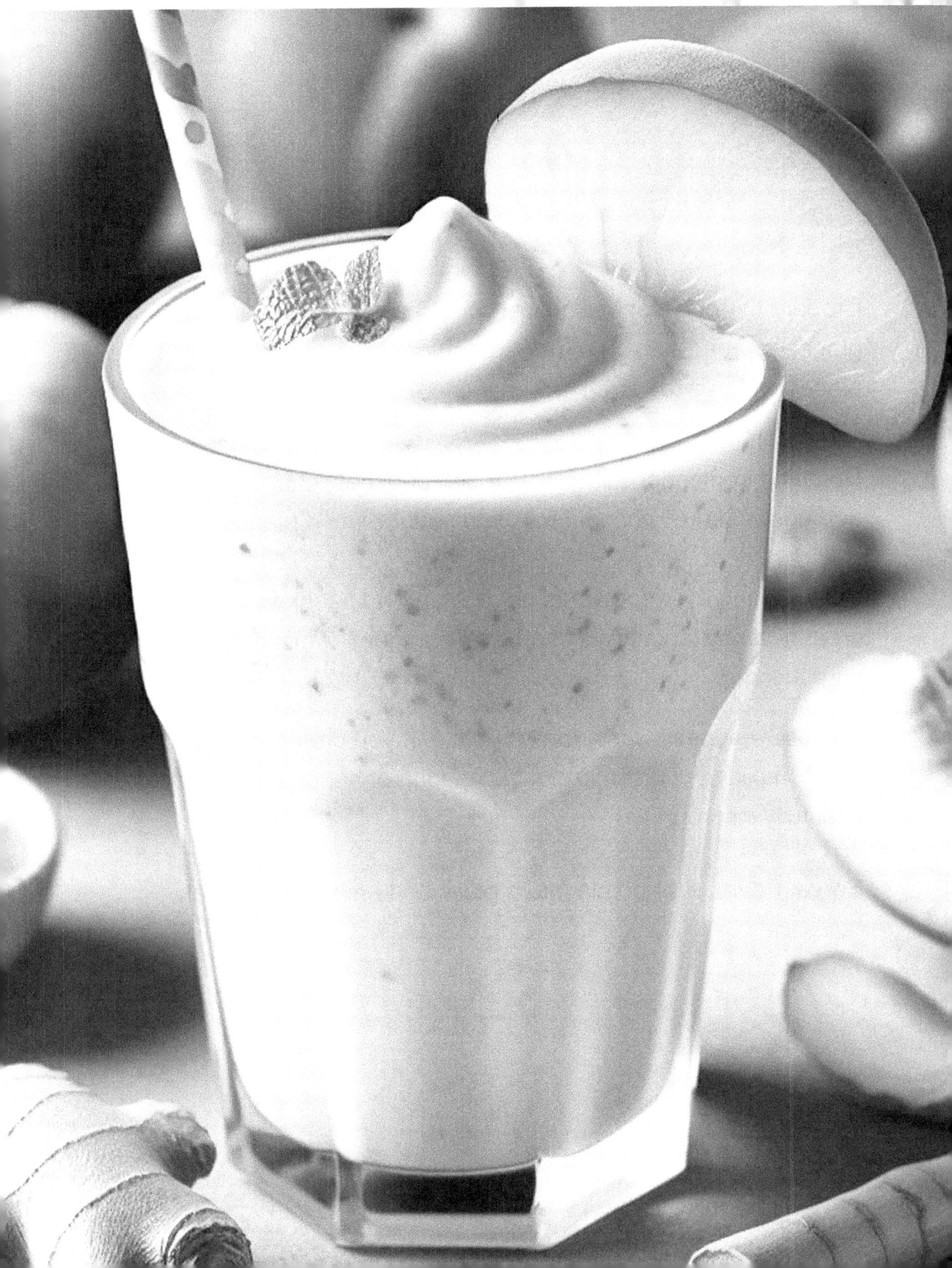

INSTRUCTIONS / DIRECTIONS

Prepare Ingredients: Make sure your frozen peaches and chopped ginger are ready. If you're using fresh peaches, cut them into small pieces and freeze them beforehand.

Combine in Blender: Place the frozen peaches, chopped fresh ginger, and unsweetened coconut milk into a high-speed blender.

Blend: Blend the ingredients on high until you achieve a smooth and creamy consistency. This should take about 1-2 minutes depending on your blender.

Adjust Sweetness: Taste the smoothie. If you prefer it sweeter and it's AIP compliant, you can add 1 tablespoon of honey and blend again until fully incorporated.

Serve: Pour the smoothie into a glass and enjoy immediately.

Hygiene practices

Wash your hands Thoroughly before handling any ingredients, with soap and warm water for at least 20 seconds to remove dirt, germs, and bacteria.

Use clean cutting boards and utensils designated for food preparation. Wash them with hot, soapy water before and after use to prevent cross-contamination.

Rinse fresh fruits and vegetables under cold, running water to remove dirt, pesticides, and bacteria. Use a brush to scrub firm produce like carrots, ginger, and turmeric to ensure thorough cleaning.

For ingredients like carrots, ginger, and turmeric, peel off the outer skin if desired. This can further reduce potential contaminants on the surface.

Use clean, filtered water for washing produce and preparing beverages. Avoid using water that may be contaminated or unsafe for consumption.

Store fresh ingredients in clean, dry containers or refrigerate them if necessary to maintain freshness and prevent spoilage.

Discard any ingredients that appear spoiled, moldy, or damaged. Use fresh, high-quality ingredients for the best flavor and nutritional value.

Clean and sanitize your blender or juicer according to the manufacturer's instructions after each use to prevent bacterial growth and ensure food safety.

Keep raw ingredients separate from cooked or ready-to-eat foods to prevent cross-contamination. Wash hands, utensils, and surfaces thoroughly after handling raw ingredients.

A Family Recipe

These recipes are designed to be AIP-friendly, avoiding common allergens and inflammatory ingredients while focusing on nutrient-dense, healing foods. Feel free to create your own recipes from the list below and give it a name of your choosing.

JUICES

Green Healing Juice: Cucumber, celery, kale, green apple, and lemon.

Anti-Inflammatory Carrot Juice: Carrot, ginger, turmeric, and apple.

Gut Health Juice: Cabbage, cucumber, green apple, and mint.

Detox Beet Juice: Beet, carrot, cucumber, and lemon.

Energy Boost Juice: Spinach, celery, green apple, and lemon.

Immune Support Juice: Orange, carrot, ginger, and lemon.

Hydration Juice: Watermelon, cucumber, and mint.

Cleansing Juice: Celery, parsley, green apple, and lemon.

Digestive Aid Juice: Fennel, cucumber, green apple, and mint.

Zesty Green Juice: Romaine lettuce, cucumber, lime, and ginger.

Refreshing Melon Juice: Honeydew melon, cucumber, and mint.

Tropical Green Juice: Pineapple, cucumber, kale, and mint.

Citrus Sunrise Juice: Orange, grapefruit, and carrot.

Sweet Green Juice: Pear, spinach, cucumber, and lemon.

Berry Bliss Juice: Strawberry, cucumber, and mint.

Red Power Juice: Beet, apple, carrot, and ginger.

Cool Mint Juice: Cucumber, celery, green apple, and mint.

Spicy Carrot Juice: Carrot, ginger, and turmeric.

Summer Refresh Juice: Watermelon, cucumber, and lime.

Nutrient Boost Juice: Kale, cucumber, green apple, and lemon.

Berry Citrus Juice: Blueberry, orange, and cucumber.

Sunshine Juice: Mango, carrot, and ginger.

Tart Green Juice: Green apple, celery, and lime.

Vitality Juice: Romaine lettuce, cucumber, and lemon.

Ginger Pear Juice: Pear, cucumber, and ginger.

SMOOTHIES

Berry Coconut Smoothie: Blueberry, coconut milk, and spinach.

Green Detox Smoothie: Kale, cucumber, avocado, and coconut water.

Pineapple Mint Smoothie: Pineapple, mint, and coconut water.

Avocado Citrus Smoothie: Avocado, orange, and spinach.

Tropical Smoothie: Mango, pineapple, and coconut milk.

Carrot Cake Smoothie: Carrot, coconut milk, and cinnamon.

Berry Kale Smoothie: Strawberry, kale, and coconut milk.

Melon Mint Smoothie: Honeydew melon, mint, and coconut water.

Peach Ginger Smoothie: Peach, ginger, and coconut water.

Green Apple Smoothie: Green apple, spinach, and coconut milk.

Beet Berry Smoothie: Beet, blueberry, and coconut water.

Cucumber Melon Smoothie: Cucumber, cantaloupe, and coconut water.

Spiced Pumpkin Smoothie: Pumpkin puree, coconut milk, and cinnamon.

Tropical Green Smoothie: Pineapple, kale, and coconut water.

Sweet Potato Pie Smoothie: Sweet potato, coconut milk, and cinnamon.

Berry Beet Smoothie: Strawberry, beet, and coconut water.

Minty Melon Smoothie: Watermelon, mint, and coconut milk.

Citrus Green Smoothie: Orange, spinach, and avocado.

Pineapple Ginger Smoothie: Pineapple, ginger, and coconut water.

Creamy Avocado Smoothie: Avocado, coconut milk, and lime.

Zesty Berry Smoothie: Raspberry, lemon, and coconut milk.

Cucumber Lime Smoothie: Cucumber, lime, and coconut water.

Tropical Beet Smoothie: Beet, mango, and coconut milk.

Peach Basil Smoothie: Peach, basil, and coconut water.

Berry Citrus Blast Smoothie: Blueberry, orange, and coconut milk.